CARDIAC ARRHYTHMIAS: SELF-LEARNING

CARDIAC ARRHYTHMIAS: SELF-LEARNING

Companion Volume to Manual of Cardiac Arrhythmias

by

Edward K. Chung, M.D.,F.A.C.P.,F.A.C.C.

Professor of Medicine
Jefferson Medical College of
Thomas Jefferson University
and
Director of the Heart Station and
Attending Physician (Cardiologist)
Thomas Jefferson University Hospital
Philadelphia, Pa. 19107

Fellow, American College of Cardiology
Former Governor for West Virginia, American College of Cardiology
Fellow, American College of Physicians
Member, American Federation for Clinical Research
Member, American Medical Association
Member, World Congress of Cardiology
Member, Asian Pacific Congress of Cardiology
Member, International Congress of Electrocardiology
Member, Pennsylvania Medical Society
Member, Philadelphia County Medical Society
Member, Korean Medical Association

Editorial Board Member for
Cardiology,
The Journal of Electrocardiology,
Primary Cardiology,
Cardiology Clinics,
and
Hospital Physicians

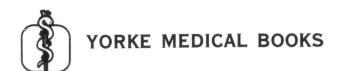

YORKE MEDICAL BOOKS

CARDIAC ARRHYTHMIAS SELF-LEARNING

Printed in the United States of America

First Edition
First Printing

International Standard Book Number: 0-914316-46-X

Library of Congress Catalog Number: 85-040840

CARDIAC ARRHYTHMIAS: SELF-LEARNING

by

Edward K. Chung, M.D., F.A.C.P., F.A.C.C.

Professor of Medicine
Jefferson Medical College
Thomas Jefferson University
and
Director of The Heart Station
Attending Physician (Cardiologist)
Thomas Jefferson University Hospital
Philadelphia, Pa. 19107

To
My Wife, Lisa
and
To Our Children, Linda and Christopher

Contents

Preface

This book, entitled *Cardiac Arrhythmias: Self Learning*, includes 200 cases showing common cardiac arrhythmias which are frequently encountered in our medical practice. Thus, this book is intended to be a companion volume to my book *Manual of Cardiac Arrhythmias*, which has been published very recently by the same publisher.

Each case describes a short case history to aid in the interpretation of the ECG tracing. The reverse side of each page gives a full analysis of the interpretation of the tracing so that the reader can assess his or her ECG diagnosis. In the majority of cases, 3 simultaneous ECG leads (leads V_1, II and V_5) recorded by 3-channel ECG equipment, are shown for the accurate diagnosis. In addition to the ECG diagnosis, the pertinent clinical significance and the therapeutic approach are included in many instances.

The arrangement of the text and illustrations is based upon the author's experience in teaching medical students, house staff, cardiology fellows, cardiac care nurses, and physicians with various backgrounds.

The unique feature of this book, like all other books by the author, is a practical approach with its clinical applications which will directly assist each reader in the diagnosis and management of his or her patient. The author hopes that the book will be of particular value to all primary care physicians including cardiologists, internists, family physicians, and emergency room physicians, in addition to medical house staff and cardiology fellows. Medical students, cardiac care nurses, and physicians with other specialties (e.g., anesthesiologists, cardiovascular surgeons), of course, will learn about various common cardiac arrhythmias in detail by reading this book.

The secretarial duties were carried out cheerfully by Ms. Michele Church Harvey, the personal secretary to the author. Her valuable contribution is greatly appreciated. It has been my pleasure to work with the staff of the Publisher, Yorke Medical Books.

Lastly, I will always owe a deep gratitude and appreciation to my father, Il-Chun Chung, M.D., who has always offered guidance and inspiration.

Bryn Mawr, Pa.   Edward K. Chung, M.D.

Suggested Readings

CHUNG EK: *Ambulatory Electrocardiography: Holter Monitor Electrocardiography*, Heidelberg-New York, Springer-Verlag Pub., 1979.

CHUNG EK: *Artificial Cardiac Pacing, Second Edition*, Baltimore, Williams & Wilkins, 1984.

CHUNG EK: *A Clinical Manual of Cardiovascular Medicine*, Norwalk, CT, Appleton-Century-Crofts Pub., 1984.

CHUNG EK: *Fundamentals of Electrocardiography*, Baltimore, University Park Press, 1984.

CHUNG EK: *Manual of Cardiac Arrhythmias*, New York, Yorke Medical Books, 1985.

CHUNG EK: *Office Electrocardiography*, Baltimore, University Park Press, 1984.

CHUNG EK: *Principles of Cardiac Arrhythmias, Third Edition*, Baltimore, Williams & Wilkins, 1983.

CHUNG EK: *Quick Reference To Cardiovascular Diseases, Second Edition*, Philadelphia, Harper/Lippincott Co., 1983.

CHUNG EK, CHUNG LS: *Introduction To Clinical Cardiology*, Basel, Switzerland, S. Karger Pub., 1983.

FOX W, STEIN E: *Cardiac Rhythm Disturbances, A Step-By-Step Approach*, Philadelphia, Lea & Febiger Pub., 1983.

HARRISON DC: *Cardiac Arrhythmias: A Decade of Progress*, Boston, GK Hall Medical Pub., 1981.

JOSEPHSON ME, SEIDES SF: *Clinical Cardiac Electrophysiology, Techniques And Interpretations*, Philadelphia, Lea & Febiger Pub., 1979.

MARRIOTT HJL: *Practical Electrocardiography, 7th Edition*, Baltimore, Williams & Wilkins Co., 1983.

MARRIOTT HJL, CONOVER MHB: *Advanced Concepts in Arrhythmias,*, St. Louis, CV Mosby Co., 1983.

NARULA OS: *Cardiac Arrhythmias: Electrophysiology, Diagnosis And Management*, Baltimore, Williams & Wilkins Co., 1979.

SCHAMROTH L: *The Disorders of Cardiac Rhythm, Second Edition*, Oxford, Blackwell Scientific Pub., 1980.

Abbreviations

AF:	Atrial fibrillation
APC:	Atrial premature contraction
AT:	Atrial tachycardia
A-V:	Atrioventricular
A-V JEB:	A-V junctional escape beat
A-V JER:	A-V junctional escape rhythm
A-V JPC:	A-V junctional premature contraction
A-V JT:	A-V junctional tachycardia
BBBB:	Bilateral bundle branch block
BFB:	Bifascicular block
BP:	Blood pressure
BTS:	Bradytachyarrhythmia syndrome
CAD:	Coronary artery disease
CCU:	Coronary care unit
CHF:	Congestive heart failure
CNS disorders:	Central nervous system disorders
COPD:	Chronic obstructive pulmonary disease
CPR:	Cardiopulmonary resuscitation
CSS:	Carotid sinus stimulation
DC shock:	Direct current shock
DI:	Digitalis intoxication
ECG:	Electrocardiogram
IHSS:	Idiopathic hypertrophic subaortic stenosis
JEB:	Junctional escape beats
JER:	Junctional escape rhythm
JPC:	Junctional premature contraction
LBBB:	Left bundle branch block
LGL syndrome:	Lown-Ganong-Levine syndrome
LVH:	Left ventricular hypertrophy
MAT:	Multifocal atrial tachycardia
MI:	Myocardial infarction
MVPS:	Mitral valve prolapse syndrome
PAT:	Paroxysmal atrial tachycardia
RBBB:	Right bundle branch block
RVH:	Right ventricular hypertrophy
S-A:	Sino-atrial
SSS:	Sick sinus syndrome
TFB:	Trifascicular block
V-A:	Ventriculoatrial
VEB:	Ventricular escape beat
VER:	Ventricular escape rhythm
VF:	Ventricular fibrillation
VPC:	Ventricular premature contraction
VT:	Ventricular tachycardia
WPW syndrome:	Wolff-Parkinson-White syndrome

Chapter 1
AV Blocks

CASE 1

This ECG tracing was taken on a 21-year-old female with no demonstrable heart disease. She was not taking any medication, and there are no symptoms.
1. What is the cardiac rhythm diagnosis?
2. What should be the proper therapeutic approach?

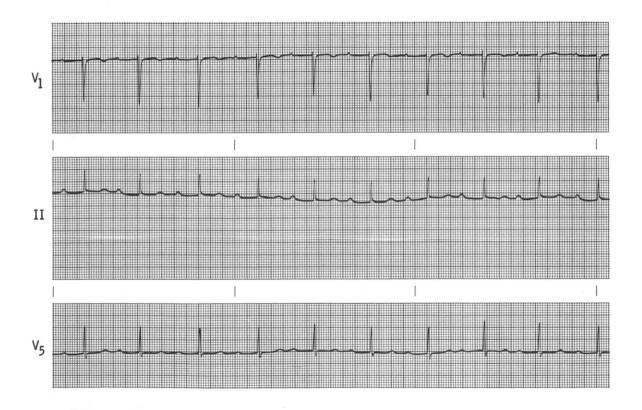

V₁

II

V₅

CASE 1: Diagnosis

The cardiac rhythm is sinus (rate: 63 beats/min) with first degree AV block (P-R interval: 0.38 second). Note that the P-R intervals are constant throughout.

It is not uncommon to observe first degree AV block in apparently healthy young individuals, and increased vagal tone is considered to be a cause. Obviously, this ECG finding is a benign arrhythmia. On the other hand, a previous inflammatory or infectious process may be the etiologic factor. At any rate, no treatment is necessary in this patient. AV block from increased vagal tone usually disappears spontaneously as the individual gets older. On rare occasions, Wenckebach AV block may be produced in young healthy individuals as a result of increased vagal tone.

First degree AV block usually represents AV nodal block (a block within the AV node).

CASE 2

A 46-year-old man with previous history of hypertension was admitted to the coronary care unit (CCU) because of chest pain. The only medication he was taking was hydrochlorothiazide 50 mg daily by mouth.

1. What is the cardiac rhythm diagnosis?
2. What is the underlying cause of this arrhythmia?
3. What is the treatment of choice?

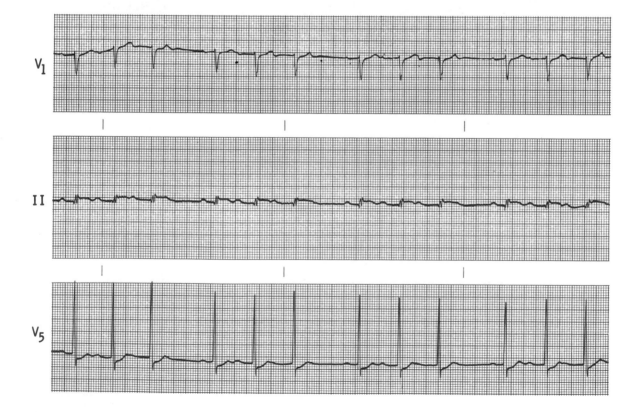

V_1

II

V_5

CASE 2: *Diagnosis*

The underlying cardiac rhythm is sinus tachycardia (atrial rate: 106 beats/min) with 4:3 Wenckebach (Mobitz type I) AV block. Note that the P-R intervals progressively lengthen, and the R-R intervals (the ventricular cycle) progressively shorten until a blocked P wave occurs. This ECG finding is a characteristic feature of Wenckebach AV block. When the AV conduction ratios are constant, as seen in this case, the cardiac rhythm exhibits a regular irregularity. Wenckebach AV block represents AV nodal block.

The direct cause of Wenckebach AV block in this patient is acute diaphragmatic (inferior) myocardial infarction (MI), and the AV block under this circumstance is nearly always transient. Thus, no treatment is necessary as long as the patient is asymptomatic from the AV block itself and the ventricular rate is well maintained (rate faster than 45–50 beats/min).

Left ventricular (LV) hypertrophy and left atrial (LA) hypertrophy are strongly suggested.

CASE 3

These ECG rhythm strips were recorded as a routine laboratory test on a 21-year-old woman with no demonstrable heart disease. She was not taking any drug.
1. What is the cardiac rhythm diagnosis?
2. What is the best therapeutic approach?

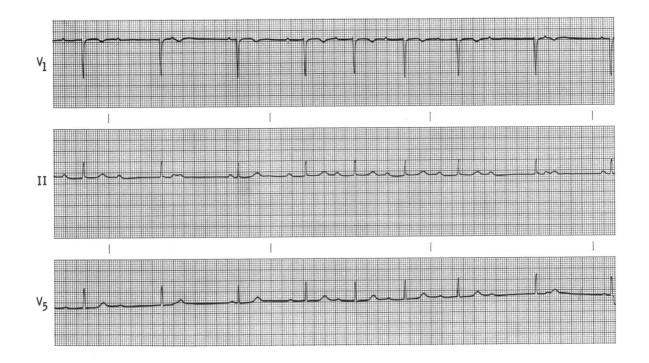

CASE 3: Diagnosis

The cardiac rhythm is sinus arrhythmia with Wenckebach (Mobitz type I) AV block and intermittent AV junctional escape beats (the 2nd, 3rd, 8th, and 9th beats). Since the progressive lengthening of the P-R intervals during Wenckebach AV conduction is minimal, inexperienced readers may not recognize the Wenckebach phenomenon readily. Intermittent AV junctional escape beats during Wenckebach AV block is not uncommon; it is a physiologic phenomenon.

Clinically, first degree or Wenckebach AV block may occur in apparently healthy youths, and, therefore, no treatment is necessary. Increased vagal tone is considered to be responsible for the production of AV block (first degree or even Wenckebach) under this circumstance.

CASE 4

This ECG tracing was taken on a 74-year-old man with coronary artery disease (CAD). He was not taking any medication and was asymptomatic.

1. What is the cardiac rhythm diagnosis?
2. What other ECG abnormalities are present?
3. Is an artificial pacemaker indicated?

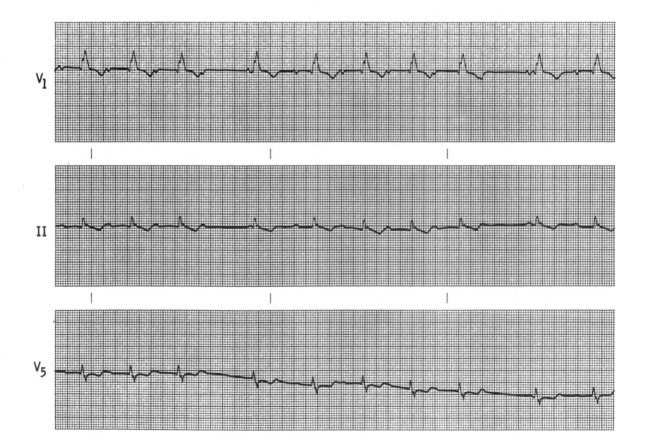

CASE 4: Diagnosis

The cardiac rhythm is sinus with Wenckebach AV block and 2 AV junctional escape beats (the 4th and 9th beats). As repeatedly emphasized, Wenckebach AV block nearly always represents AV nodal block, which is transient and self-limited in most cases. Although a combination of right or left bundle branch block (RBBB or LBBB) and second degree AV block is said to be often a manifestation of incomplete bilateral bundle branch block (infranodal block), Wenckebach AV block almost always represents AV nodal (intranodal) block. Thus, no active treatment is necessary in this patient for AV block, and artificial pacing is not indicated.

The diagnosis of RBBB is obvious, but evidence of diaphragmatic-lateral MI is not clear. However, the diagnosis of MI is obvious when the patient's 12-lead ECG is reviewed.

CASE 5

A 75-year-old woman was admitted to the CCU because of acute chest pain associated with slow heart rate. She was not taking any medication.
1. What is the cardiac rhythm diagnosis?
2. What is the underlying cause of this arrhythmia?
3. What is the proper therapeutic approach?

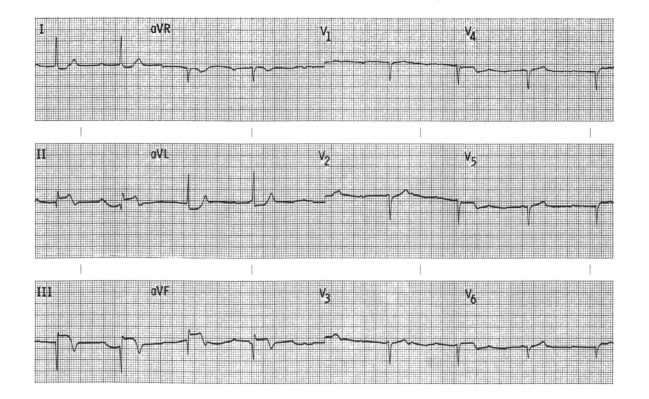

CASE 5: Diagnosis

The cardiac rhythm is sinus tachycardia (atrial rate: 108 beats/min) with AV junctional escape rhythm (ventricular rate: 53 beats/min) due to complete AV block. Note that the R-R intervals are regular and the atrial and ventricular activities are independent throughout.

The diagnosis of acute diaphragmatic MI is obvious, and complete AV block in this case is due to acute diaphragmatic MI. Under this circumstance, complete AV block represents AV nodal block, which is transient in most cases.

The therapeutic approach depends upon the presence or absence of significant hemodynamic abnormality and/or significant symptoms (e.g., syncope, near-syncope, or hypotension). By and large, a stable AV junctional escape rhythm with relatively fast ventricular rate (rate ranging from 50 to 60 beats/min) is unlikely to be associated with significant hemodynamic abnormality and/or symptoms.

Artificial pacing (usually temporary) is indicated when complete AV block in acute diaphragmatic MI is associated with significant hemodynamic abnormality and/or symptoms. When the ventricular rate in complete AV block is slower than 45 beats/min, often there are hemodynamic abnormality and/or significant symptoms. When complete AV block associated with acute diaphragmatic MI is asymptomatic and no significant hemodynamic abnormality is present, a value of artificial cardiac pacing is not certain.

In addition to acute diaphragmatic MI, the diagnosis of old anterior MI is strongly considered.

CASE 6

This ECG tracing was obtained from a 78-year-old man with a long-standing hypertension. He has been taking hydrochlorothiazide 50 mg daily by mouth for several years. He denies dizziness, near-syncope, or syncope.

1. What is the cardiac rhythm diagnosis?
2. What is the proper therapeutic approach?

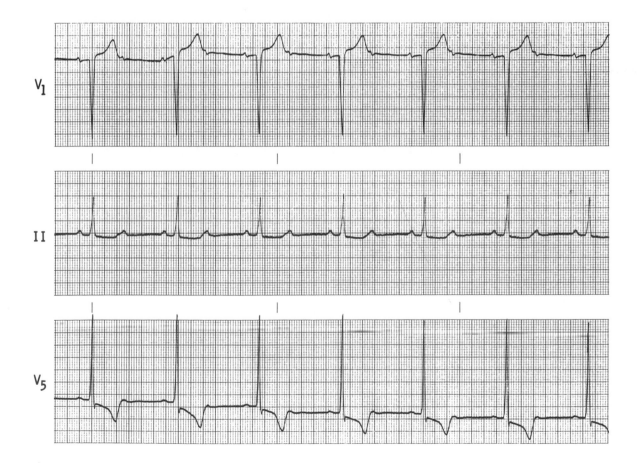

CASE 6: *Diagnosis*

The cardiac rhythm is sinus (atrial rate: 88 beats/min) with 2:1 AV block (ventricular rate: 44 beats/min). Note that every other P wave is conducted to the ventricles and the QRS complexes are normal.

When dealing with 2:1 AV block with normal QRS complexes, the site of block is in the AV node (AV nodal block) in most cases. Artificial cardiac pacing (permanent) should be strongly recommended when the AV block (even 2:1) has been a chronic conduction disturbance that is associated with significant symptoms (e.g., syncope or near-syncope) and/or the ventricular rate is constantly slower than 45 beats/min.

On the other hand, electrophysiologic study should be performed when 2:1 AV block is a chronic AV block but no significant symptom is present to determine the site of AV block. If the block is distal to the AV node (infranodal block), permanent artificial pacing should be strongly considered. When 2:1 AV block is associated with LBBB or RBBB, the block is usually due to infranodal block, in which permanent artificial pacing is considered to be indicated. Holter monitor ECG is valuable in documenting possible, more advanced forms of AV block.

The diagnosis of left ventricular hypertrophy can be made without any difficulty.

CASE 7

This ECG tracing was obtained from a 31-year-old woman. She was not taking any medication and was not complaining of any symptom other than irregular and slow pulse.
1. What is the cardiac rhythm diagnosis?
2. What is the proper therapeutic approach?

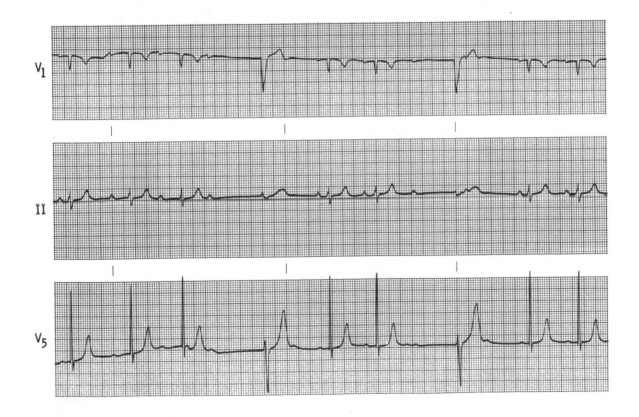

CASE 7: *Diagnosis*

The cardiac rhythm is sinus arrhythmia (atrial rate: 70 beats/min) with Wenckebach AV block and 2 ventricular escape beats (the 4th and 7th beats).

There are two reasons for the occurrence in Wenckebach AV block of ventricular escape beats instead of the expected AV junctional escape beats. One reason is that the site of AV block is distal to the His bundle (infra-His block). Another reason is the diseased AV node that is unable to produce the expected escape impulses in AV nodal block.

Electrophysiologic study is highly recommended in order to determine the site of the AV block. If the block is distal to the AV node or His bundle, permanent artificial pacing should be considered. Holter monitor ECG is valuable in documenting any other cardiac arrhythmias (possible areas of advanced or complete AV block). If the block is found to be within the AV node from the electrophysiologic evaluation and the patient is asymptomatic, she should be observed as a long-term evaluation to assess the progression of AV block. Occurrence of ventricular escape beats in Wenckebach AV block is rather unusual.

CASE 8

A 54-year-old man was evaluated at the cardiac clinic because
cardiac arrhythmia. He was not taking any medication, althoug
was found to be mildly hypertensive. He denied any significant car
symptom.
1. What is the cardiac rhythm diagnosis?
2. What is the proper therapeutic approach?

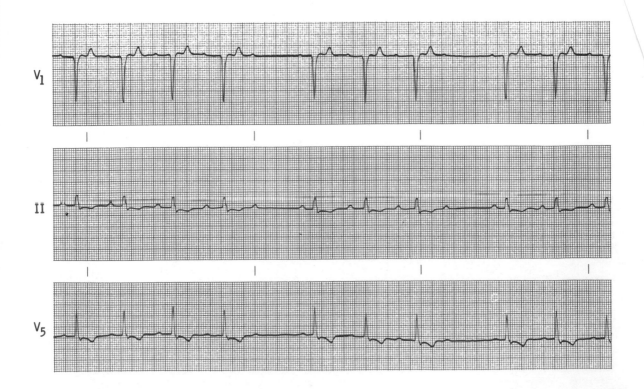

CASE 8: *Diagnosis*

The cardiac rhythm is sinus (atrial rate: 70 beats/min) with Wenckebach AV block. The AV conduction ratios vary in this ECG tracing.

No active treatment is necessary for Wenckebach AV block as long as the patient is asymptomatic and the ventricular rate is reasonably fast (greater than 50 beats/min).

The diagnosis of left ventricular hypertrophy is suggested.

The patient should be observed at the cardiac clinic periodically for possible development of more advanced AV block or a new symptom (e.g., syncope or near-syncope). Holter monitor ECG will be valuable in this case for the same purpose.

CASE 9

These ECG rhythm strips were recorded from a 70-year-old woman who complained of dizziness and near-syncope for several months. She was not taking any drug.
1. What is the cardiac rhythm diagnosis?
2. What is most likely the underlying disease process in the production of this arrhythmia?
3. What is the proper therapeutic approach?

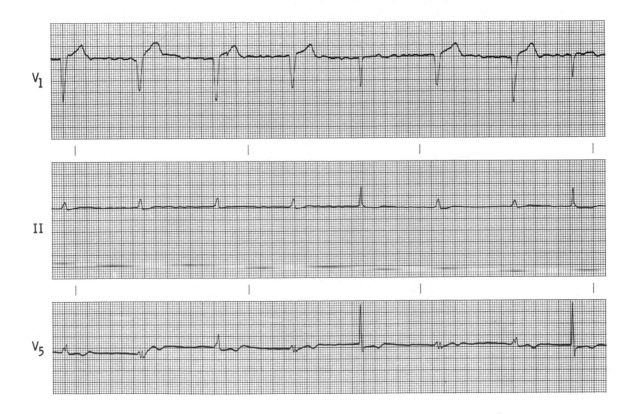

CASE 9: *Diagnosis*

The underlying cardiac rhythm is AF, but the ventricular rate is relatively slow (rate: 45 beats/min) and regular in most areas. In addition, the configuration of the QRS complexes during a regular ventricular cycle is broad and bizarre. Thus, the final cardiac rhythm diagnosis is AF with intermittent ventricular escape (idioventricular) rhythm due to advanced AV block. Note that there are occasional ventricular fusion beats (e.g., the 3rd beat).

Failure of the AV junctional escape beats to appear in this tracing is due either to the diseased AV node or to a block distal to the AV node. At any rate, the underlying disease process responsible for the production of this arrhythmia is most likely advanced sick sinus syndrome (SSS).

Permanent artificial pacing is recommended for all patients with symptomatic and/or advanced SSS. Advanced SSS is often manifested by chronic AF with advanced AV block, as seen in this case. In many patients with advanced SSS, sinus node and AV node are diseased altogether.

CASE 10

A 48-year-old man developed a slow heart rhythm soon after surgical replacement of the aortic valve for aortic insufficiency. Before the surgery, he had normal sinus rhythm.
1. What is the cardiac rhythm diagnosis?
2. What is the proper therapeutic approach?

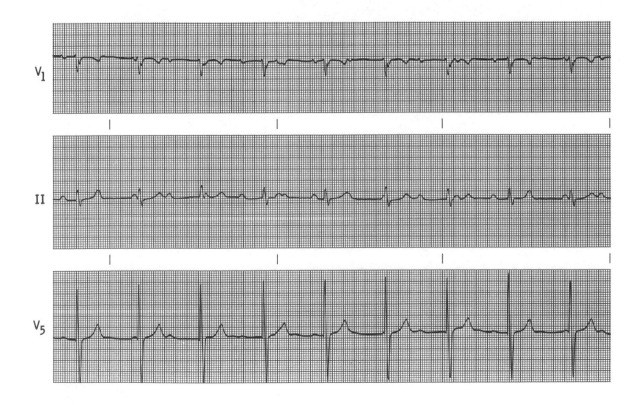

V₁

II

V₅

CASE 10: *Diagnosis*

The cardiac rhythm is sinus (atrial rate: 94 beats/min) with AV junctional escape rhythm (ventricular rate: 53 beats/min) due to complete AV block. The site of the AV block is considered to be within the AV node in this patient.

Permanent artificial pacing should be considered if the AV block persists (for 2–3 weeks) postoperatively, even if the patient is asymptomatic from complete AV block itself. Postoperative (surgery-induced) complete AV block may be transient or permanent depending upon the damage on the conduction system by the surgery and the presence or absence of the preexisting AV conduction disturbance.

CASE 11

This ECG tracing was recorded on a 73-year-old woman as a part of her annual medical checkup. She was not taking any drug and was asymptomatic except for occasional dizziness.
1. What is the cardiac rhythm diagnosis?
2. What is the most likely underlying disease process to produce this arrhythmia?
3. What is the proper therapeutic approach?

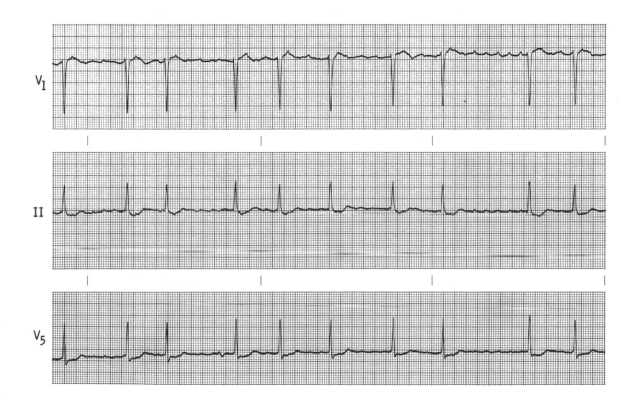

CASE 11: Diagnosis

The underlying cardiac rhythm is atrial flutter–fibrillation, but the ventricular rate is relatively slow (rate: 50–60 beats/min) as a result of advanced AV block. The underlying disease process for the production of this arrhythmia is most likely advanced SSS.

Permanent artificial pacing is recommended for all patients with symptomatic (e.g., syncope or near-syncope) or advanced SSS. Advanced SSS often produces chronic AF, flutter–fibrillation (a mixed form between atrial fibrillation and flutter), or flutter with advanced AV block causing slow irregular ventricular cycle.

CASE 12

An 89-year-old man was evaluated at the cardiac clinic because of slow heart rate. His wife stated that he had been taking digoxin 0.25 mg once and quinidine 0.3 g 4 times daily by mouth for several months. He complained of weakness and anorexia.

1. What is the cardiac rhythm diagnosis?
2. What is the proper therapeutic approach?

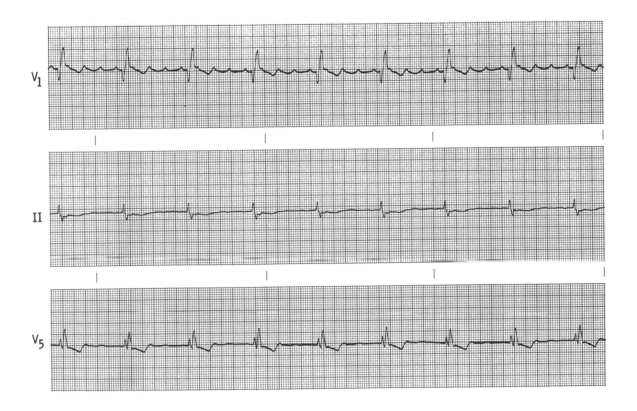

CASE 12: *Diagnosis*

The cardiac rhythm is atrial flutter (atrial rate: 212 beats/min) with 4:1 AV block (ventricular rate: 53 beats/min). Note that the ventricular cycle is precisely regular but every 4th flutter wave is conducted to the ventricles.

The atrial flutter cycle is much slower than usual (the usual atrial flutter rate ranges from 250 to 350 beats/min) in this patient because of the quinidine effect. Remember that the atrial refractory period is often increased by quinidine or quinidinelike drugs, such as procainamide. Advanced AV block (4:1 AV block in this case) is produced by digitalis.

It has been well documented that the serum digoxin level often rises when quinidine is administered at the same time, and, therefore, digoxin toxicity is easily produced. Thus, digoxin dosage has to be reduced whenever quinidine is given simultaneously.

This patient was found to have an elevated digoxin level in the serum (3.2 ng/ml) as a result of digoxin toxicity. Both digoxin and quinidine were discontinued in this case, and later only digoxin was restarted. An indication for quinidine for this patient was not found.

The diagnosis of RBBB is obvious.

CASE 13

An 84-year-old woman was admitted to the CCU because a heart attack was suspected. She was not taking any medication.
1. What is the cardiac rhythm diagnosis?
2. What is most likely to be the cause of this arrhythmia?
3. What is the best therapeutic approach?

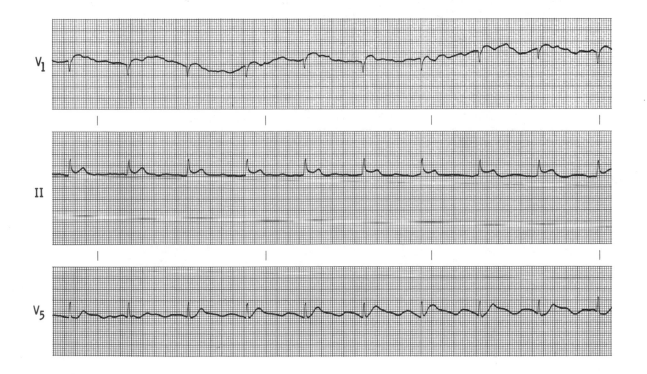

CASE 13: Diagnosis

The underlying cardiac rhythm is AF, but the R-R intervals are regular and the ventricular rate is relatively slow (ventricular rate: 58 beats/min). Thus, the final rhythm diagnosis is AF with AV junctional escape rhythm (rate: 58 beats/min) due to complete AV block.

The direct cause of complete AV block in this patient is acute diaphragmatic MI (pathologic Q waves with S-T segment elevation in leads III and aVF—not shown here). It is well documented that AV block of any degree is very common in acute diaphragmatic MI as a result of impairment of the blood supply to the AV node. Remember that the AV nodal blood supply commonly arises from the right coronary artery, and acute diaphragmatic MI is frequently caused by right coronary artery occlusion. Under this circumstance, the site of AV block is within the AV node (AV nodal block), and, therefore, AV block is transient in most patients.

As long as the ventricular rate is relatively rapid (faster than 50 beats/min) and stable in complete AV block, there is usually no significant hemodynamic abnormality or symptom (e.g., syncope or near-syncope). Thus, no active treatment is necessary. Temporary artificial pacing is indicated, however, when the patient is symptomatic from AV block itself or significant hemodynamic abnormality is produced. In this case, the ventricular rate is generally slow (rate: less than 40–45 beats/min) and unstable.

Permanent artificial pacing should be considered when complete AV block persists more than 2–3 weeks under this clinical circumstance (very rare).

CASE 14

Cardiac consultation was requested on a 79-year-old woman because she was found to have slow heart rhythm associated with frequent episodes of dizziness and near-syncope for several months. She was not taking any drug.

1. What is the cardiac rhythm diagnosis?
2. What ECG abnormalities are present?
3. What is the proper therapeutic approach?

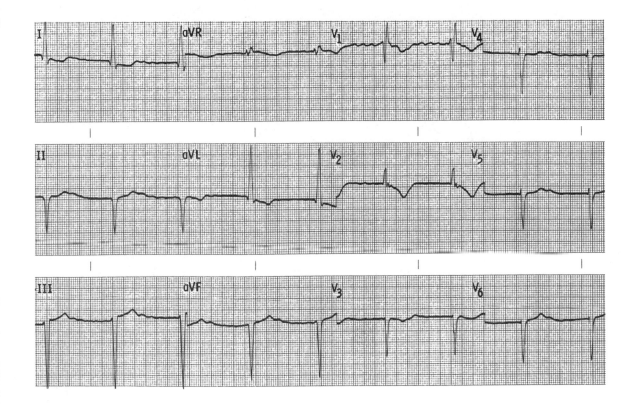

CASE 14: Diagnosis

The cardiac rhythm diagnosis is AF with AV junctional escape rhythm (ventricular rate: 48 beats/min) due to complete AV block. Note that the ventricular cycle is regular throughout, indicating that the atrial and ventricular activities are independent.

Other ECG abnormalities include bifascicular block (BFB) consisting of RBBB and left anterior hemiblock (QRS axis: -65 degree) associated with anterolateral MI (loss of R wave amplitude in leads V_{3-6}). In addition, left ventricular hypertrophy is diagnosed.

Permanent artificial pacing is strongly recommended for chronic complete AV block, especially when the patient is symptomatic and the ventricular rate is relatively slow. The underlying disease process in this patient is most likely to be advanced SSS. It has been shown that various conduction disturbances (e.g., RBBB, AV block) often coexist with advanced SSS, and the underlying rhythm is AF in many cases.

CASE 15

A 70-year-old woman was examined at the cardiac clinic for evaluation of her cardiac status. She had been in relatively good health other than mild hypertension. She was not taking any medication. Her only complaint was weakness associated with occasional dizziness.

1. What is the cardiac rhythm diagnosis?
2. What is the proper therapeutic approach?

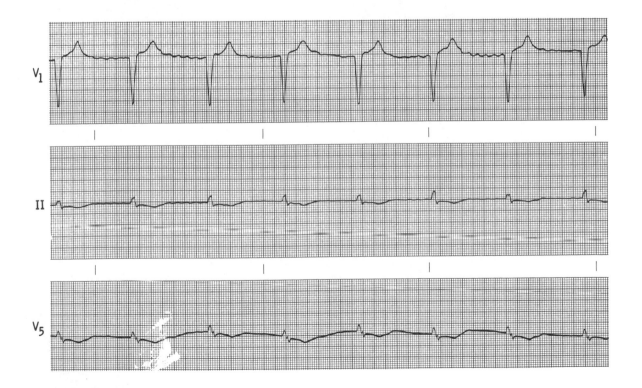

CASE 15: Diagnosis

The underlying cardiac rhythm is AF, but the ventricular cycle is regular with relatively slow ventricular rate (rate: 44 beats/min). Thus, there is complete AV block. The QRS configuration demonstrates LBBB pattern. It is uncertain whether the escape rhythm represents AV junctional escape rhythm with preexisting LBBB or ventricular escape rhythm when no other ECG tracings (taken previously in this case) are available in order to determine the presence or absence of LBBB. Judging from the relatively fast ventricular rate (rate above 30–40 beats/min) in this patient, the rhythm diagnosis is most likely AF with AV junctional escape rhythm due to complete AV block associated with LBBB.

Permanent artificial pacing is recommended for chronic complete AV block. The underlying disease process in this patient is most likely advanced SSS.

CASE 16

A 54-year-old man was admitted to the intermediate cardiac care unit for evaluation of his several episodes of fainting or near-syncope for several months. The patient found that his pulse rate was very slow at least several months previously. He was not taking any medication.

1. What is the cardiac rhythm diagnosis?
2. What is the proper therapeutic approach?

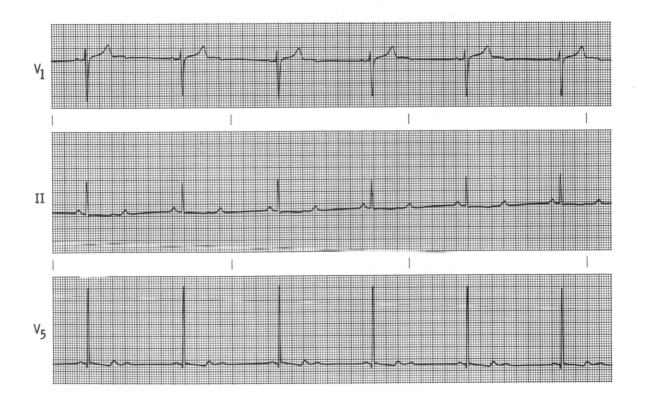

CASE 16: *Diagnosis*

The cardiac rhythm reveals sinus rhythm (atrial rate: 76 beats/min) with 2:1 AV block. Note that every other P wave is blocked and the QRS complexes are normal (narrow). When dealing with 2:1 AV block with normal QRS complexes, the site of the block is often within the AV node, and 2:1 AV block in this circumstance is usually a variant of Wenckebach AV block.

However, because of significant symptoms (syncope or near-syncope) and the chronic nature of the AV block, Holter monitor ECG was obtained, which shows frequent areas demonstrating complete AV block with intermittent ventricular escape rhythm (not shown here). Furthermore, electrophysiologic study confirmed that the block was distal to the AV node (infranodal block).

A permanent artificial pacemaker was implanted in this patient, and his symptoms did not recur after pacing.

The diagnosis of left ventricular hypertrophy is obvious.

CASE 17

A 27-year-old woman was seen in the cardiologist's office because of very slow pulse rate since her birth. She was relatively asymptomatic except for slight exercise intolerance since early childhood. She was not taking any medication.
1. What is the cardiac rhythm diagnosis?
2. What is the proper therapeutic approach?

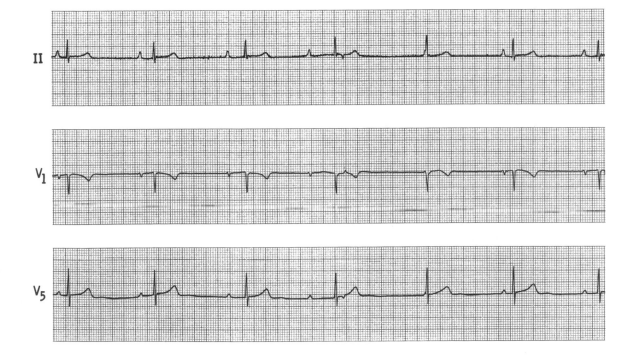

CASE 17: Diagnosis

This ECG tracing exhibits sinus bradycardia (atrial rate: 43 beats/min) with AV junctional escape rhythm (ventricular rate: 38 beats/min) due to complete AV block. All sinus P waves are independent to the QRS complexes, but there is a retrograde P wave following the 4th QRS complex. This retrograde P wave represents an atrial echo (reciprocal) beat due to a reentry phenomenon, so that there is a relationship—although momentary—between the atria and the ventricles. Consequently, the rhythm disorder reveals incomplete AV dissociation.

A permanent artificial pacemaker is required for all patients with congenital complete AV block because the block is irreversible. Complete AV block may or may not be associated with other congenital cardiac anomalies. All patients with congenital complete AV block become significantly symptomatic as they get older.

Chapter 2
Intraventricular Block

CASE 18

This ECG tracing was obtained from a 73-year-old man with no demonstrable heart disease. He was asymptomatic and was not taking any medication.

1. What is the ECG diagnosis?

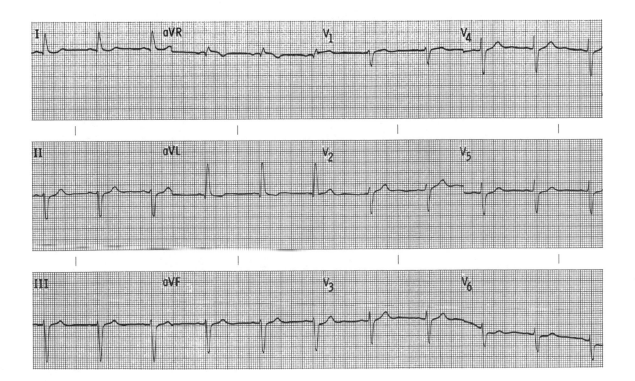

CASE 18: Diagnosis

The cardiac rhythm is sinus with a rate of 60 beats/min. The diagnosis of left anterior hemiblock can be made without any difficulty on the basis of marked left axis deviation of the QRS complexes (QRS axis: −65 degrees). In addition, the QRS duration is relatively broad (QRS interval: 0.12 second) so that diffuse (nonspecific) intraventricular block is present.

The final diagnosis of this ECG tracing is left anterior hemiblock with diffuse intraventricular block. No treatment, of course, is necessary for this ECG finding.

The diagnostic criteria of left anterior hemiblock are as follows:

1. Marked left axis deviation of the QRS complexes (−45 to −90)
2. Small q wave in lead I and small r wave in lead III
3. Little or no prolongation of QRS interval
4. No evidence of other factors responsible for the production of left axis deviation

CASE 19

A 66-year-old woman with a long-standing mild hypertension was seen at the hypertensive clinic for a periodic medical checkup. She was asymptomatic, and the only medication she has been taking was hydrochlorothiazide 50 mg daily by mouth.

1. What is the ECG diagnosis?

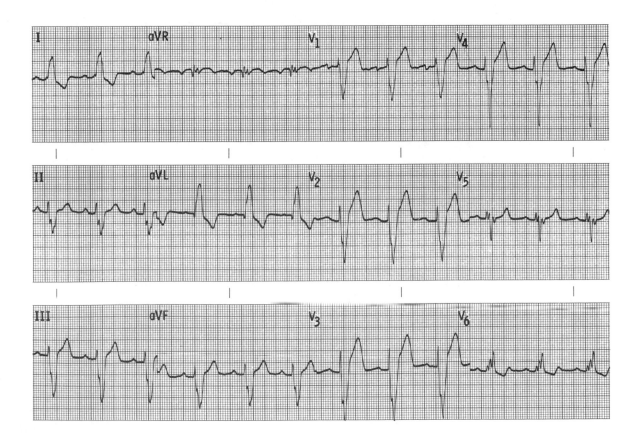

CASE 19: Diagnosis

The cardiac rhythm is sinus, with a rate of 72 beats/min. It is obvious that the QRS complexes are broad and bizarre because of LBBB.

The most important ECG finding of LBBB is absence of physiologic (septal) q waves in the left precordial leads as a result of abnormal septal activation. Because of delayed activation of the left ventricle, the QRS complexes in the left precordial leads usually exhibit RR′ (M-shaped) or broad upright R waves associated with secondary T waves (biphasic or inverted T waves). The secondary T waves are not symmetrically inverted.

In addition, left atrial enlargement is suggested.

Clinically, LBBB is very common in patients with a long-standing hypertension, and the left ventricle is usually hypertrophied.

CASE 20

An 81-year-old woman was admitted to the CCU because of chest pain of several hours in duration. She was not taking any medication.
1. What is the ECG diagnosis?
2. What is the proper therapeutic approach?

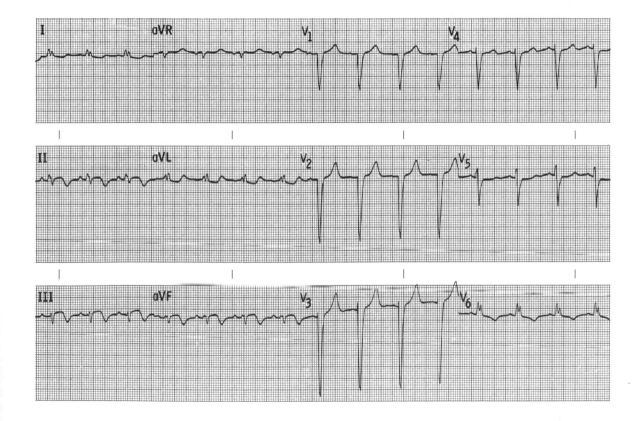

CASE 20: Diagnosis

The cardiac rhythm is sinus, with a rate of 88 beats/min. The diagnosis of LBBB can be entertained on this ECG tracing without any difficulty (see Case 19).

However, the T waves are deeply and symmetrically inverted in leads II, III, and aVF associated with S-T segment elevation. These T wave abnormalities are the primary T wave change and not the secondary T wave change. Thus, the diagnosis of acute diaphragmatic MI is strongly considered. Later, acute MI is confirmed by serial serum enzyme study with myocardial scan.

Remember that pure LBBB is associated with the secondary T wave change (see Case 19) and the T waves are not symmetrically inverted.

Prophylactic artificial pacing is usually not indicated for acute or preexisting LBBB or RBBB associated with acute MI. The QRS amplitude in the limb leads is small, indicating low voltage.

CASE 21

This ECG tracing was taken on a 77-year-old man with known CAD. He had suffered from a heart attack 6 months previously, and his recovery was uneventful.
1. What is the ECG diagnosis?
2. What is the proper therapeutic approach?

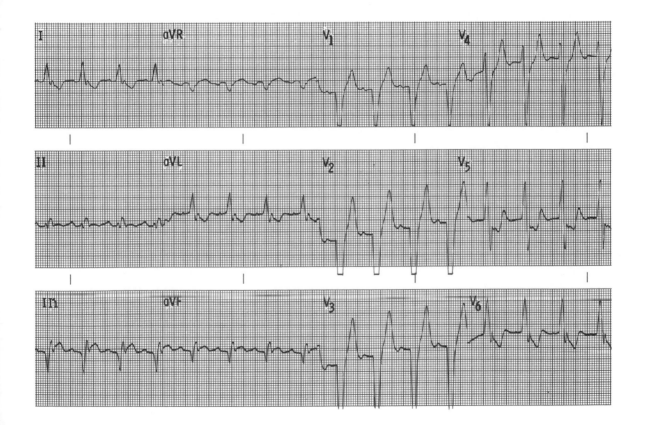

CASE 21: Diagnosis

The cardiac rhythm is sinus, with a rate of 95 beats/min. The diagnosis of LBBB is readily made (see Case 19).

Another obvious ECG abnormality is evidence of diaphragmatic (inferior) MI (pathologic Q waves in leads III and aVF). Ventricular aneurysm may be suspected when the S-T segment elevation persists following an episode of acute MI. However, S-T segment elevation not uncommonly continues for many weeks, months, years, or even indefinitely after acute MI with no evidence of ventricular aneurysm.

No active treatment is necessary for LBBB associated with diaphragmatic MI (acute or old).

CASE 22

Cardiology consultation was requested on a 22-year-old man who had had a heart murmur since early childhood. He had been relatively asymptomatic, but a form of congenital heart disease was suspected by his family physician.
1. What is the ECG abnormality?
2. What is the most likely underlying cardiac disease?

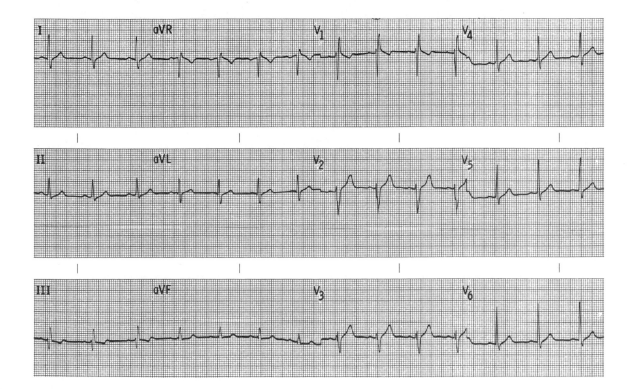

CASE 22: *Diagnosis*

The cardiac rhythm is sinus arrhythmia, with rate ranging from 72 to 84 beats/min. The diagnosis of incomplete RBBB can be made without any difficulty on the basis of RR' in lead V_1, with persisting and slightly broad S waves in the left precordial leads. The total duration of the QRS complex is not more than 0.10 second. These ECG abnormalities are due to slightly delayed right ventricular activation as a result of incomplete RBBB.

As far as the underlying heart disease responsible for the production of this ECG abnormality (incomplete RBBB) is concerned, the most likely congenital cardiac anomaly is atrial septal defect. It can be said that RBBB (more commonly the incomplete form) is found in more than 95% of patients with atrial septal defect. In other words, the diagnosis of atrial septal defect is very remote when the ECG fails to demonstrate RBBB.

Less commonly, RBBB may be observed in other congenital cardiac anomalies, including tetralogy of Fallot, ventricular septal defect, and Ebstein's anomaly.

CASE 23

This ECG tracing was taken on a 68-year-old man during his annual medical checkup. He had been apparently healthy with no demonstrable heart disease.

1. What is the ECG diagnosis?
2. What is the proper therapeutic approach?

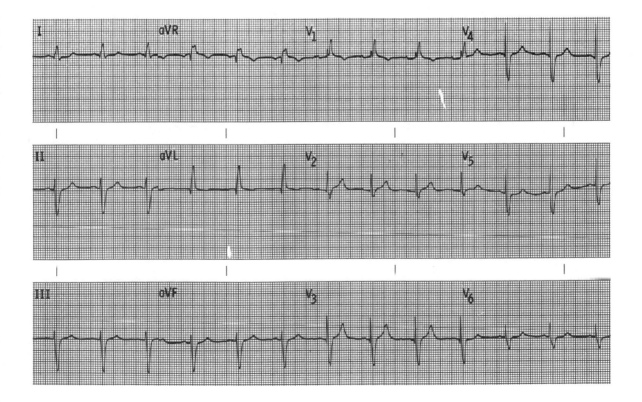

CASE 23: Diagnosis

The cardiac rhythm is sinus, with a rate of 75 beats/min. This ECG tracing shows BFB, which consists of RBBB and left anterior hemiblock (QRS axis: −75 degree). BFB is, of course, the most common form of incomplete bilateral bundle branch block (BBBB).

The diagnostic criteria of BBBB are summarized as follows:

Diagnostic Criteria of Bilateral Bundle Branch Block
(Bifascicular Block and Trifascicular Block)

1. RBBB with left anterior hemiblock
2. RBBB with left posterior hemiblock
3. Alternating LBBB and RBBB
4. LBBB or RBBB with first degree or second degree AV block
5. LBBB or RBBB with prolonged (>55 msec) H-V interval
6. LBBB on one occasion and RBBB on another occasion
7. Mobitz type II AV block
8. Any combination of the above findings
9. Complete AV block with ventricular escape (idioventricular) rhythm

No treatment is necessary for asymptomatic BFB. When the patient develops any symptom (e.g., syncope or near-syncope) related to bradyarrhythmia (as manifestations of advanced BBBB), the Holter monitor ECG and/or electrophysiologic study should be performed in order to document such arrhythmias for possible consideration of permanent artificial cardiac pacing.

CASE 24

A 76-year-old man was seen in the emergency room because of palpitations associated with anxiety. He was not taking any medication and denied any episode of syncope, near-syncope, or chest pain.

1. What is the ECG diagnosis?
2. What is the proper therapeutic approach?

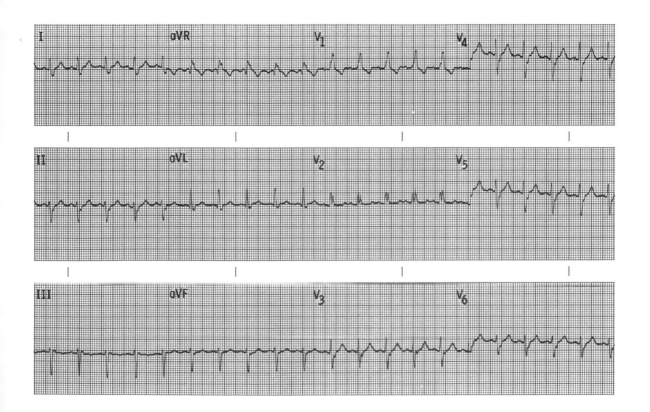

CASE 24: Diagnosis

The cardiac rhythm is sinus tachycardia with a rate of 120 beats/min. The diagnosis of BFB consisting of RBBB and left anterior hemiblock (QRS axis: −80 degrees) is made readily according to the diagnostic criteria described previously (see Case 23).

No treatment is indicated for asymptomatic BFB. Mild to even marked sinus tachycardia is not uncommon when the patient is nervous or anxious because of various reasons. When significantly rapid sinus tachycardia (rate above 120 beats/min) persists at resting state, however, the underlying causes (e.g., anemia, hyperthyroidism, occult malignancy, fever) should be investigated.

CASE 25

An 89-year-old man was admitted to the CCU because of chest pain of a few hours in duration. He was not taking any medication.
1. What is the ECG diagnosis?

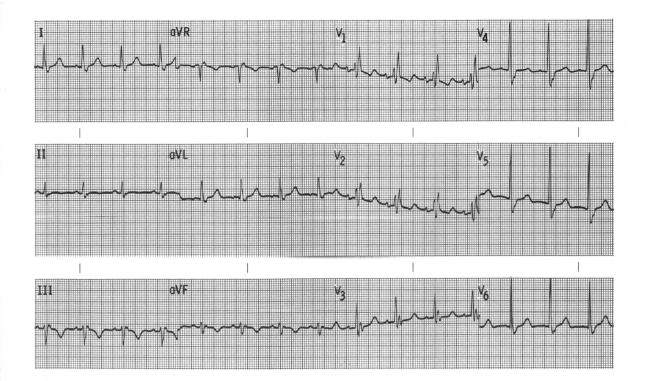

CASE 25: Diagnosis

The cardiac rhythm is sinus, with a rate of 85 beats/min. RBBB is obvious, but symmetrically inverted T waves in leads III and aVF are not due to RBBB. Diaphragmatic (inferior) myocardial ischemia is diagnosed. In addition, left ventricular hypertrophy is suggested by the voltage criteria. The clinical diagnosis of this patient is angina pectoris. The evidence of acute MI is not found in this patient by serial ECGs and serum enzyme study.

CASE 26

A 76-year-old woman with a history of angina pectoris was admitted to the CCU because of increasing severity of chest pain of 4–5 hours in duration. Sublingual nitroglycerine (3 tablets) was ineffective for chest pain.
1. What is the ECG diagnosis?
2. What is the proper therapeutic approach?

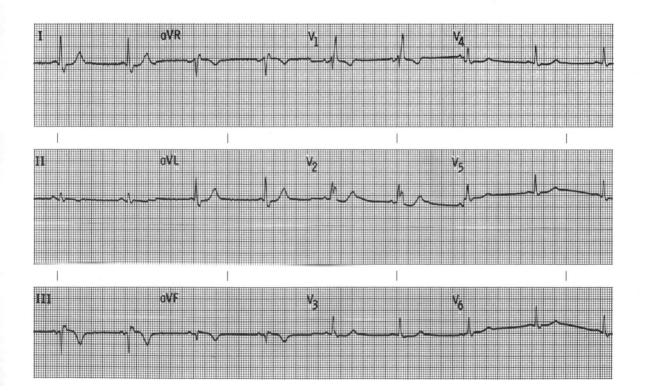

CASE 26: *Diagnosis*

The cardiac rhythm is sinus bradycardia, with a rate of 50 beats/min. There are 2 ECG abnormalities, which include RBBB and recent diaphragmatic MI. It should be noted that the diagnosis of diaphragmatic MI is not difficult in the presence of RBBB. The reason for this is that RBBB causes an abnormal *terminal* conduction delay, whereas diaphragmatic MI causes an abnormality in the *initial* portion of the QRS complex (pathologic Q waves). In other words, the initial activation of the ventricles is not altered by the RBBB.

The patient requires the usual acute coronary care for acute MI. Prophylactic artificial pacing is not indicated for acute or preexisting RBBB in patients with acute MI regardless of the location of MI. Likewise, no treatment is necessary for mild asymptomatic sinus bradycardia. When sinus bradycardia is marked (rate: usually slower than 40–45 beats/min), atropine may be tried and is usually effective. Temporary artificial pacing is only rarely indicated for severe sinus bradycardia.

CASE 27

A 55-year-old obese woman was brought to the emergency room because a heart attack was suspected. She was not taking any medication.
1. What is the ECG diagnosis?
2. What is the proper therapeutic approach?

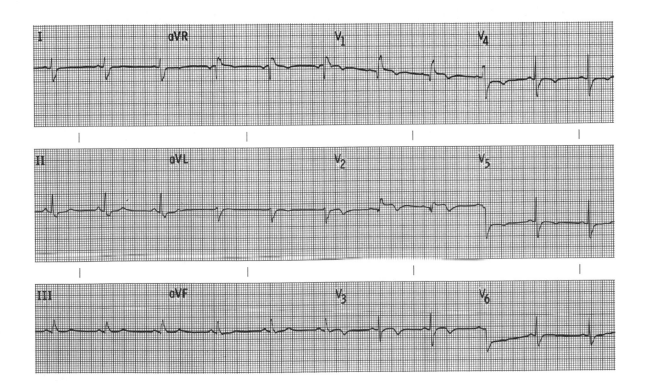

CASE 27: *Diagnosis*

The cardiac rhythm is sinus, with a rate of 62 beats/min. The diagnosis of acute anteroseptal MI is readily made on the basis of abnormal Q waves in leads V_{1-2} associated with marked S-T segment elevation and inverted T waves in all precordial leads. Another ECG abnormality is BFB, which consists of RBBB and left posterior hemiblock (QRS axis: +120 degree).

It is generally agreed that prophylactic artificial pacing is indicated for BFB of acute onset, usually due to acute anteroseptal MI and extensive anterior MI. It should be emphasized that various forms of intraventricular conduction disturbances are relatively common as a result of acute anteroseptal MI because the Purkinje system is frequently damaged by the MI. The damage to the Purkinje system is often permanent under this circumstance. Indications for permanent artificial pacing in patients with acute MI will be discussed later (see Case 28).

The diagnostic criteria of left posterior hemiblock are as follows:

Diagnostic Criteria of Left Posterior Hemiblock

1. Marked right axis deviation (+105 to +180 degrees)
2. Small r wave in lead I and small q wave in lead III
3. Little or no prolongation of QRS interval
4. No evidence of other factors responsible for right axis deviation (true or pseudo)

CASE 28

A 60-year-old man was transferred from another hospital for further management of his acute coronary event. This ECG tracing was taken on admission to the CCU (about 7–8 hours after the onset of acute chest pain). Review of his hospital record (from another hospital) revealed that he had had a transient complete AV block and BFB consisting of RBBB and left anterior hemiblock on other occasions (during 5–6 hours of hospitalization at another hospital).

1. What is the ECG diagnosis?
2. What is the proper therapeutic approach?

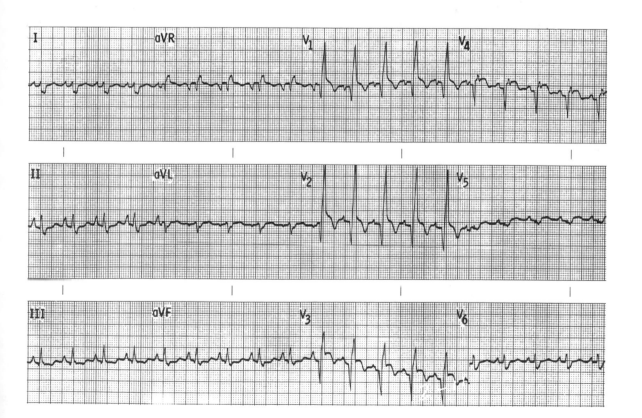

CASE 28: Diagnosis

The cardiac rhythm is sinus tachycardia, with a rate of 110 beats/min. The ECG abnormalities include acute extensive anterior MI associated with BFB consisting of RBBB and left posterior hemiblock (QRS axis: +120 degree). Because of acute BFB on admission, a temporary artificial pacemaker was inserted.

Later, a permanent artificial pacemaker was implanted because the patient had intermittent complete AV block before his transfer from another hospital. He had also had left anterior hemiblock with RBBB on other occasions. When all ECG abnormalities are analyzed together, this patient unequivocally demonstrates incomplete trifascicular block (TFB) as a result of acute extensive anterior MI.

It is generally agreed that permanent artificial pacing is recommended for all patients with acute anterior MI who develop complete AV block even transiently as a manifestation of incomplete TFB (see Case 23).

The ECG diagnosis of P-pulmonale is made on the basis of peaking and tall P waves in leads II, III, and aVF. Acute pulmonary embolism was suspected, and further diagnostic studies confirmed the diagnosis (by lung scan).

CASE 29

This ECG tracing was taken on an 86-year-old man who was admitted to the CCU because of a recent heart attack.
1. What is the ECG diagnosis?
2. What is the proper therapeutic approach?

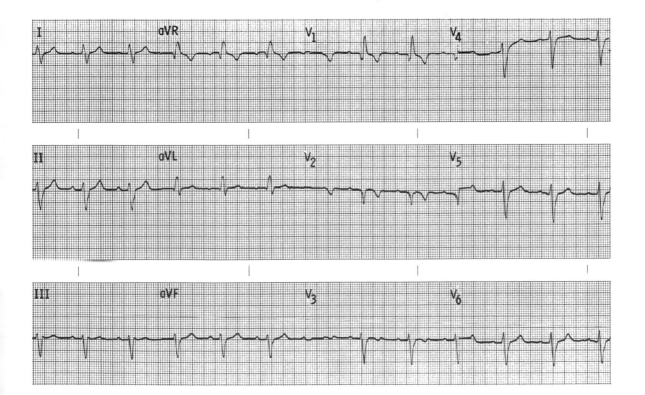

CASE 29: *Diagnosis*

The cardiac rhythm is sinus, with a rate of 74 beats/min. The ECG tracing reveals recent anteroseptal MI associated with BFB, consisting of RBBB and left anterior hemiblock (QRS axis: −90 degree).

Prophylactic temporary artificial pacing is indicated for acute BFB as a result of recent anteroseptal MI.

CASE 30

A 42-year-old man with a history of a heart attack 6 months previously was seen at the cardiac clinic for follow-up evaluation. He had been relatively asymptomatic, except for occasional angina.
1. What is the ECG diagnosis?
2. What is the proper therapeutic approach?

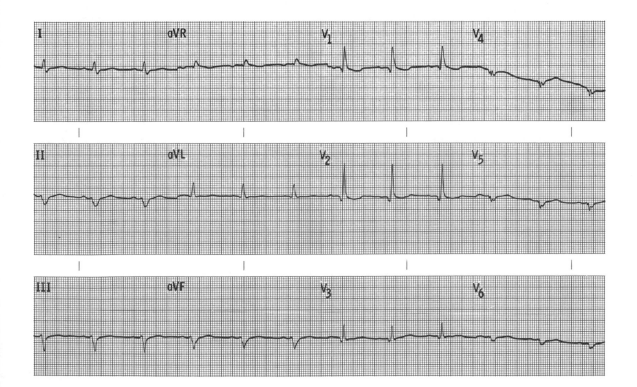

CASE 30: Diagnosis

The cardiac rhythm is sinus, with a rate of 67 beats/min. The evidence of old extensive anterior MI is obvious in this ECG tracing (abnormal Q waves in all precordial leads). In addition, there is BFB, which consists of RBBB and left anterior hemiblock (QRS axis: −85 degree).

The exact onset of BFB in this patient is uncertain, although it was probably a complication of anterior MI that occurred 6 months previously. At any rate, artificial cardiac pacing is not indicated for old or preexisting BFB.

CASE 31

This ECG tracing was taken on a 56-year-old man with CAD. He had suffered from a heart attack 3 months previously, and his recovery was uneventful.

1. What is the ECG diagnosis?

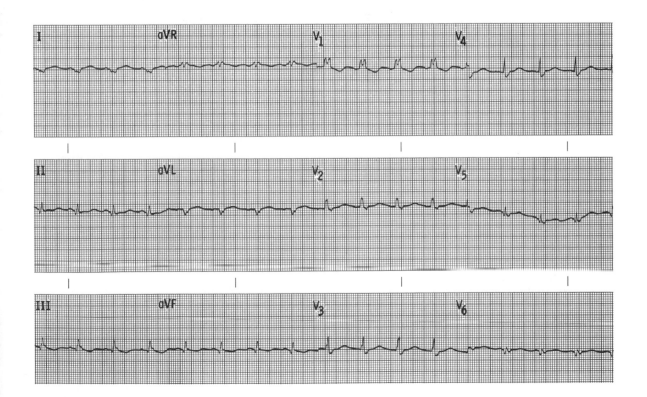

CASE 31: *Diagnosis*

The cardiac rhythm is sinus with a rate of 94 beats/min. The diagnosis of RBBB can be made without any difficulty, but some readers may not recognize a coexisting posterior MI. It should be noted that the initial R wave in lead V_1 is taller than expected, and there is complete loss of posterior force as a result of posterior MI. In addition, the diagnosis of diaphragmatic-lateral MI is established on the basis of pathologic Q waves in leads II, III, aVF, and V_{5-6}. Furthermore, Q-S waves in leads I and aVL indicate high lateral MI.

Thus, the final diagnosis of this ECG tracing is diaphragmatic posterolateral MI associated with RBBB. The QRS amplitude is generally small in most leads indicating "low voltage". The term, "low voltage", is used when the sum of QRS amplitude (both positive and negative components) in leads I, II, and III is 15 mm or less. Low voltage of the QRS complex is relatively common in patients with massive MI.

CASE 32

A 61-year-old woman was seen in the medical clinic at a periodic medical checkup.
1. Wha is the ECG diagnosis?
2. What is most likely the underlying disorder?

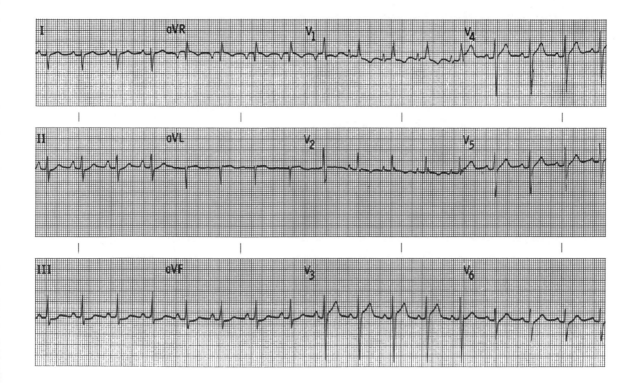

CASE 32: Diagnosis

The underlying cardiac rhythm is sinus with a rate of 95 beats/min. The P waves are peaked and tall in inferior leads, and this ECG finding is termed "P-pulmonale" because it is often found in advanced chronic obstructive pulmonary disease (COPD). The diagnosis of right ventricular hypertrophy is established on the basis of right axis deviation of the QRS complexes (QRS axis: +120 degree) associated with incomplete RBBB.

When dealing with the above-mentioned ECG abnormalities (P-pulmonale, right ventricular hypertrophy with incomplete RBBB), the underlying disorder is most commonly advanced COPD.

CASE 33

This ECG tracing was obtained from a 57-year-old woman with chronic congestive heart failure (CHF). A form of cardiomyopathy was considered to be the underlying heart disease. She has been taking digoxin 0.25 mg daily by mouth for several months.
1. What is the ECG diagnosis?

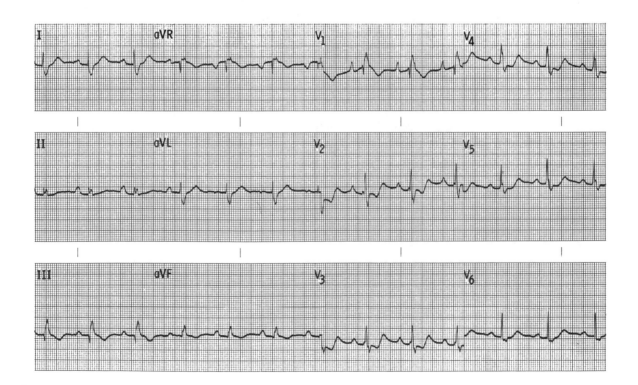

CASE 33: Diagnosis

The cardiac rhythm is sinus (rate: 72 beats/min) with first degree AV block (P-R interval: 0.22 second). The P waves are broad and tall in many leads, indicative of biatrial hypertrophy. The diagnosis of RBBB can be established without any difficulty. In addition, right ventricular hypertrophy is strongly considered because the QRS axis reveals a tendency to right axis deviation (exact QRS axis cannot be determined precisely on this tracing).

In addition, a possibility of diaphragmatic MI is raised because of borderline pathologic Q waves in inferior leads.

These ECG abnormalities as mentioned above are not uncommon in patients with advanced cardiomyopathy (various types). Pseudo MI pattern is also relatively common under this circumstance.

CASE 34

A 72-year-old man who had undergone surgical repair for atrial septal defect several years previously was seen at the cardiac clinic for an annual checkup.

1. What is the ECG diagnosis?

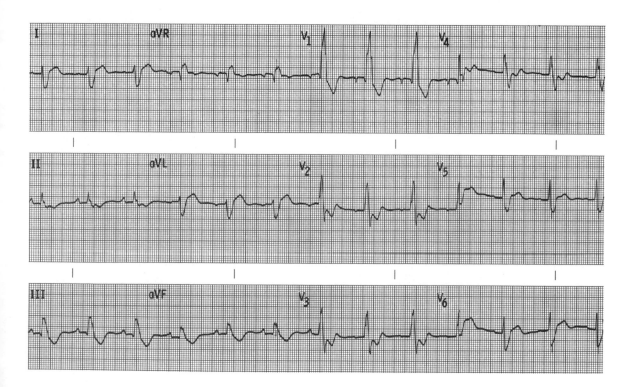

CASE 34: Diagnosis

The cardiac rhythm is sinus (rate: 70 beats) with first degree AV block (P-R interval: 0.22 second). BFB, which consists of RBBB and left posterior hemiblock (QRS axis: +135 degrees), is obvious. Whenever there is right axis deviation of the QRS complex in the presence of RBBB, however, right ventricular hypertrophy should always be considered.

The P waves are peaked in the inferior leads, suggestive of right atrial hypertrophy. The term "P-congenitale" is used to describe right atrial hypertrophy due to any form of congenital heart disease.

In addition, old diaphragmatic (inferior) MI is a remote possibility.

The above-mentioned ECG abnormalities (RBBB with normal or abnormal QRS axis, P-congenitale, and first degree AV block) are common in patients with atrial septal defect. Even after surgical repair for atrial septal defect, the ECG abnormalities often persist.

CASE 35

This ECG tracing was recorded from a 71-year-old man with known CAD.
1. What is the ECG diagnosis?
2. What is the proper therapeutic approach?

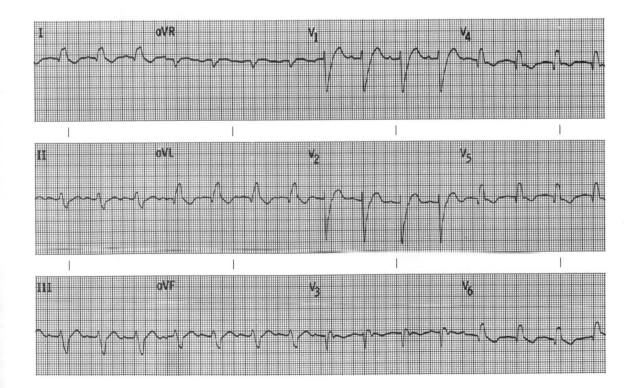

CASE 35: *Diagnosis*

The cardiac rhythm is sinus (rate: 86 beats/min) with first degree AV block (P-R interval: 0.22 second). LBBB is superficially simulated, but the broad QRS complexes in this ECG tracing are due to left anterior hemiblock with diffuse (nonspecfic) intraventricular block. The diagnosis of lateral MI (including the involvement of high lateral wall) is established without any difficulty on the basis of pathologic Q waves in leads I, aVL, and V_{4-6}. In addition, left atrial hypertrophy is suggested.

Various forms of intraventricular block are relatively common in patients with MI, especially when anterior wall (including lateral wall) is involved. No active treatment is indicated for hemiblocks or diffuse intraventricular block associated with MI.

CASE 36

A 67-year-old man with a previous history of a heart attack was seen at the cardiologist's office for follow-up evaluation.

1. What is the ECG diagnosis?

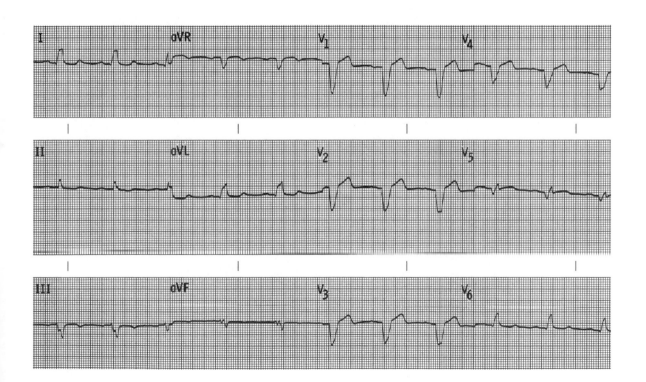

CASE 36: Diagnosis

The cardiac rhythm is sinus (rate: 62 beats/min) with first degree AV block (P-R interval: 0.22 second). Extensive anterior MI is diagnosed on the basis of Q-S waves, or embryonic R waves, in leads V_{1-4}, with Q waves in leads V_{5-6}. The QRS complexes are broad because of diffuse (nonspecific) intraventricular block. This ECG finding closely mimics LBBB. Remember that a pure LBBB is manifested by a loss of septal (physiologic) q waves in the left precordial leads (see Case 19).

In addition, the diagnosis of left atrial hypertrophy is considered.

CASE 37

This ECG tracing was taken on a 69-year-old man with diffuse cardiomegaly.

1. What is the ECG diagnosis?

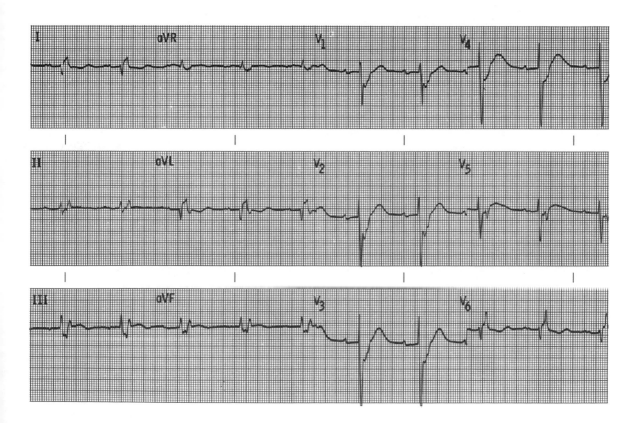

CASE 37: Diagnosis

The cardiac rhythm is sinus bradycardia (rate: 57 beats/min) with first degree AV block (P-R interval: 0.28 second). The diagnosis of left atrial hypertrophy is made on the basis of broad and notched P waves in many limb leads, with a deep and broad negative component of P waves in leads V_{1-3}.

The striking ECG abnormality is extremely broad and bizarre QRS complexes. This ECG finding is diagnostic of LBBB, but it is rather atypical in configuration.

It has been shown that various forms of cardiomyopathy are frequently associated with atypical LBBB or RBBB. All cardiac chambers are shown to be markedly hypertrophied in this patient, and his cardiomyopathy is proven to be idiopathic.

CASE 38

A 66-year-old woman with cardiomyopathy was examined at the cardiac clinic as a periodic medical checkup.
1. What is the ECG diagnosis?

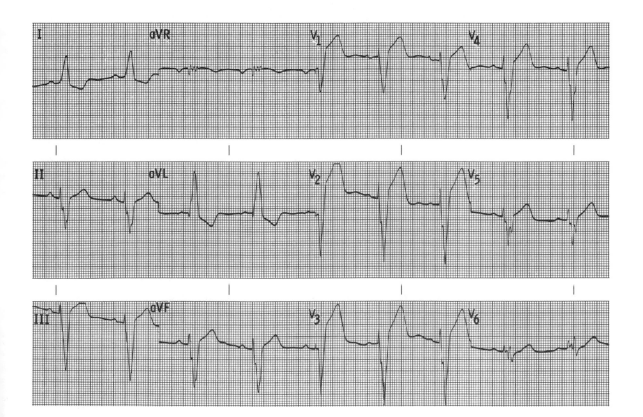

CASE 38: Diagnosis

The cardiac rhythm is sinus bradycardia (rate: 55 beats/min). The diagnosis of LBBB as well as left atrial hypertrophy is established without much difficulty. These ECG findings are similar to those shown in Case 37, but LBBB in this tracing is closer to the typical (pure) form. Remember that LBBB may be associated with normal QRS axis or left axis deviation.

CASE 39

This ECG tracing was obtained from a 74-year-old woman with a previous history of a heart attack. Initially, frequent ventricular premature contractions (VPCs) were diagnosed erroneously.

1. What is the ECG diagnosis?

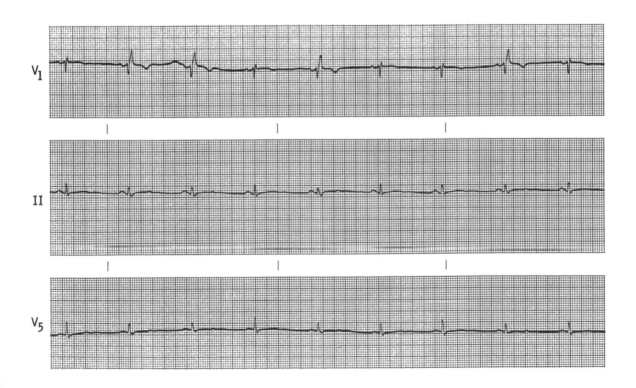

CASE 39: Diagnosis

The cardiac rhythm is sinus bradycardia with a rate of 54 beats/min. On superficial examination, the ECG abnormality appears to be frequent VPCs, but the correct diagnosis is intermittent RBBB, which occurs independent of the cardiac cycle. Therefore, this finding is termed "rate-independent" RBBB. By close observation, incomplete RBBB can be recognized in the remaining beats. Accordingly, this tracing demonstrates intermittent complete and incomplete RBBB. Intermittent RBBB is insignificant clinically, but the ECG finding may be misdiagnosed as ventricular ectopy. The diagnosis of old diaphragmatic MI is established on 12-lead ECG (not shown here).

CASE 40

A 70-year-old man with known CAD visited the cardiac clinic for follow-up evaluation.

1. What is the ECG diagnosis?

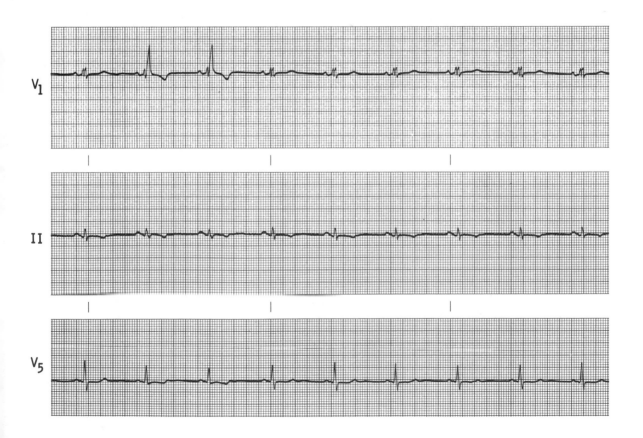

CASE 40: Diagnosis

The cardiac rhythm is sinus bradycardia with a rate of 58 beats/min. It is obvious that complete and incomplete RBBB occur intermittently, unrelated to the cardiac cycle (see Case 39). The diagnosis of posterior MI is strongly considered on the basis of a relatively tall initial R wave in lead V_1 with upright T wave. Remember that the T wave is either inverted or biphasic in lead V_1 when dealing with pure RBBB (see Case 39).

CASE 41

Cardiac consultation was requested because of the ECG abnormality shown here.
1. What is the ECG diagnosis?

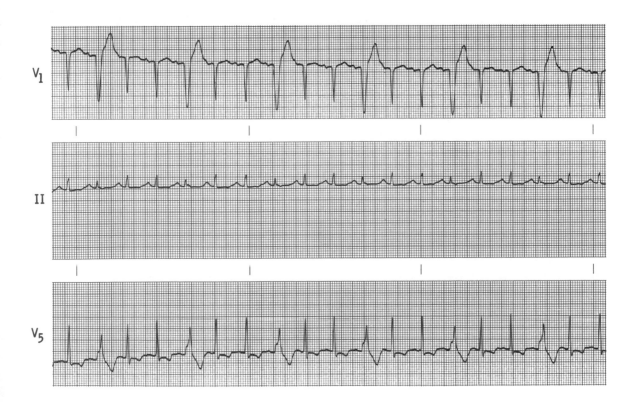

CASE 41: Diagnosis

The cardiac rhythm is sinus tachycardia with a rate of 118 beats/min. It should be noted that broad QRS complexes appear on every 3rd beat. This ECG finding is intermittent LBBB, which closely simulates frequent VPCs causing ventricular trigeminy. Since LBBB occurs with a regular rhythmicity, it is considered to be rate dependent.

CASE 42

This ECG tracing was taken on a 60-year-old man with a previous history of MI.

1. What is the ECG diagnosis?

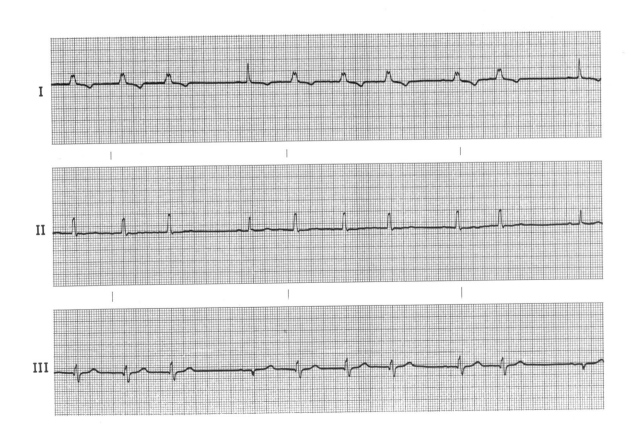

CASE 42: Diagnosis

The cardiac rhythm is marked sinus bradycardia (rate: 43 beats/min) and frequent atrial premature contractions (APCs) with group beats. It is apparent that there are 2 kinds of QRS complexes because of intermittent LBBB. LBBB occurs in this ECG tracing during the faster heart rate, indicating rate-dependent (more precisely "tachycardia-dependent") LBBB.

In addition, the evidence of old diaphragmatic MI is present in this ECG tracing (pathologic Q wave in lead III).

CASE 43

An 82-year-old woman was evaluated at the cardiac clinic because of slow pulse rate associated with dizziness for several months. She was not taking any medication.
1. What is the ECG diagnosis?
2. What is the proper therapeutic approach?

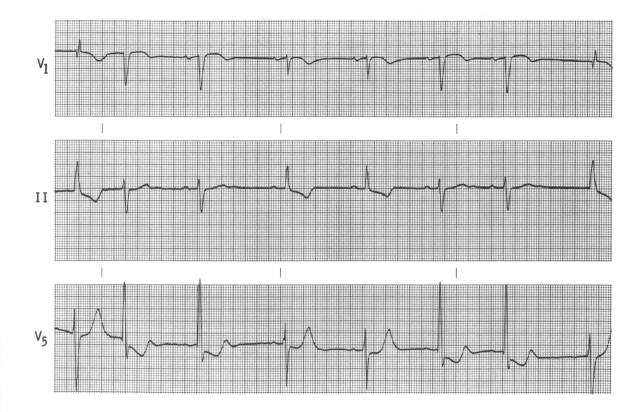

CASE 43: Diagnosis

The cardiac rhythm is sinus bradycardia (atrial rate: 45 beats/min) with first degree AV block and intermittent sinus arrest leading to occasional ventricular escape beats (the first and the last beats). In addition, there is intermittent left anterior hemiblock (the 2nd, 3rd, 6th, and 7th beats). The underlying disorder responsible for these ECG findings is most likely SSS. Permanent artificial pacemaker implantation is highly recommended.

Other ECG abnormalities include left ventricular hypertrophy and left atrial hypertrophy.

CASE 44

These ECG tracings (A, B, and C) were recorded from an 89-year-old woman. She has been relatively asymptomatic except for such nonspecific complaints as weakness and dizziness. She has been taking digoxin 0.25 mg daily by mouth for several months.
1. What is the ECG diagnosis of each ECG tracing?
2. What is the proper therapeutic approach?

A

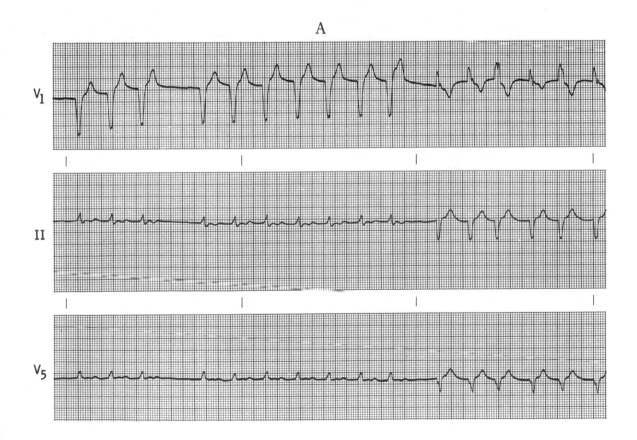

V_1

II

V_5

B

C

CASE 44: Diagnosis

Tracing A

The underlying cardiac rhythm is AF (ventricular rate: 110 beats/min), but there is intermittent nonparoxysmal AV junctional tachycardia (regular R-R intervals in some areas). It is obvious that there are 2 forms of QRS complexes. That is, LBBB occurs intermittently with BFB, consisting of RBBB and left anterior hemiblock.

Tracing B

This tracing taken a few hours later exhibits BFB, which consists of RBBB and left anterior hemiblock (QRS axis: −90 degrees). The cardiac rhythm is essentially unchanged (AF with intermittent nonparoxysmal AV junctional tachycardia).

Tracing C

This tracing was recorded several hours later and reveals LBBB. The cardiac rhythm is essentially unchanged.

When these findings are analyzed together, this patient demonstrates the best example of incomplete TFB (incomplete BBBB).

The Holter monitor ECG should be obtained in order to determine whether this patient develops intermittent complete BBBB leading to intermittent ventricular escape rhythm. When intermittent complete BBBB (see Case 23) is documented, permanent artificial pacemaker implantation is definitely indicated.

Chapter 3
Sinus Arrhythmias

CASE 45

A 73-year-old woman was seen at medical clinic as an annual medical checkup. She was apparently healthy and not taking any medication.
1. What is the cardiac rhythm diagnosis?
2. What is the proper therapeutic approach?

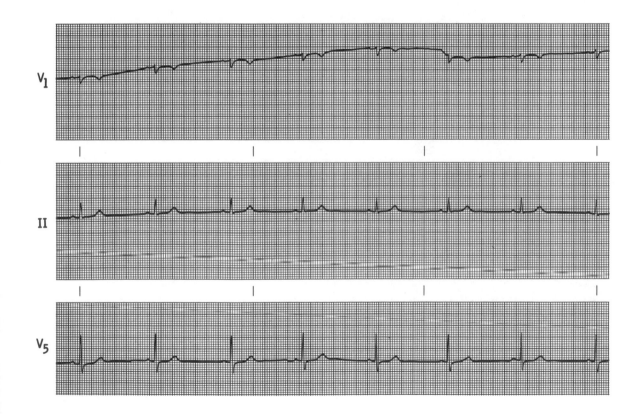

V₁

II

V₅

CASE 45: Diagnosis

The cardiac rhythm is sinus bradycardia with a rate of 48 beats/min. Although it is not absolutely necessary, the Holter monitor ECG is recommended, considering the patient's age and marked sinus bradycardia. If any evidence of advanced SSS is documented, artificial cardiac pacing should be considered. Electrophysiologic study (e.g., determination of the sinus node recovery time) is not necessary unless the Holter monitor ECG findings are very suspicious but not conclusive for the diagnosis of advanced SSS (see Case 9).

It should be noted that the earliest manifestation of SSS is sinus bradycardia, especially in elderly people, although many healthy individuals may have significant sinus bradycardia. Thus, marked sinus bradycardia may or may not be a normal finding in a given individual.

CASE 46

This ECG tracing was taken at the student health center on a 26-year-old female as a routine medical evaluation. She was found to be healthy.

1. What is the cardiac rhythm diagnosis?

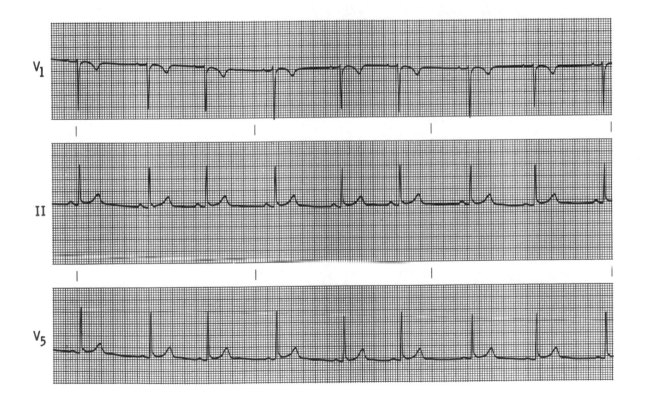

CASE 46: *Diagnosis*

The cardiac rhythm diagnosis is sinus bradycardia with sinus arrhythmia at a rate of 53–56 beats/min. This type of sinus arrhythmia is very common among healthy young individuals. Since the sinus cycle varies according to the respiratory cycle under this circumstance, the term "respiratory sinus arrhythmia" is used.

Conversely, sinus arrhythmia that is not related to the respiratory cycle is termed "nonrespiratory sinus arrhythmia." This latter form of sinus arrhythmia is relatively common in elderly people and cardiac patients. At times, marked sinus arrhythmia may be an early sign of SSS.

Respiratory sinus arrhythmia in young people is, of course, a physiologic phenomenon.

CASE 47

A 30-year-old man was admitted to the surgical service because of a possible diagnosis of acute appendicitis. This ECG tracing was taken as a part of the preoperative laboratory tests.

1. What is the cardiac rhythm diagnosis?

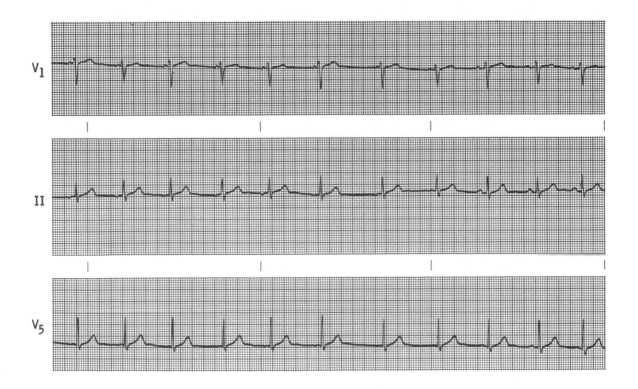

CASE 47: Diagnosis

The cardiac rhythm is sinus arrhythmia with wandering atrial pacemaker at a rate of 60–72 beats/min. It should be noted that the P wave configuration varies considerably, associated with a varying P-P cycle.

Wandering atrial pacemaker under this circumstance is considered to be an exaggerated form of sinus arrhythmia. This arrhythmia is clinically insignificant.

CASE 48

Cardiac consultation was requested for the evaluation of a some-what unusual P wave configuration. The patient was an apparently healthy 25-year-old woman with a near-term pregnancy.
1. What is the cardiac rhythm diagnosis?

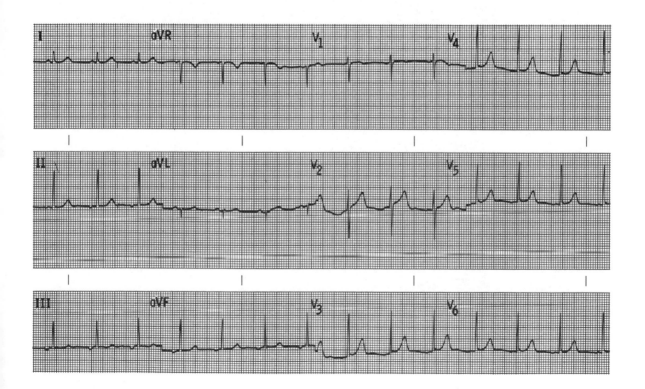

CASE 48: Diagnosis

On superficial examination, the cardiac rhythm appears to be an ordinary sinus rhythm. On close observation, however, most readers can recognize inverted P waves in leads II, III, and aVF. Since the P wave is slightly inverted in lead aVR, the P axis is measured to be −50 degrees.

According to the standard diagnostic criteria, the P wave axis of retrograde conduction is considered to be between −60 and −90 degrees. Thus, the cardiac rhythm with the P wave axis less than −60 degrees (between 0 and −60 degrees) most likely originates from the sinus node. This type of cardiac rhythm is called "sinus rhythm with left axis deviation of P waves."

As far as clinical significance is concerned, left axis deviation of the P waves may be found in apparently healthy people, although it may be an early sign of left atrial hypertrophy in some patients. In addition, left axis deviation of the P waves may be observed in individuals with pregnancy, massive ascites, or marked obesity.

CASE 49

These cardiac rhythm strips were taken on a 30-year-old woman who complained of several episodes of syncope and near-syncope. Successful surgical repair for atrial septal defect was performed approximately 10 years ago, and the recovery was uneventful at that time. Leads II-a and II-b are continuous. She was not taking any drug.
1. What is the cardiac rhythm diagnosis?
2. What is the proper therapeutic approach?

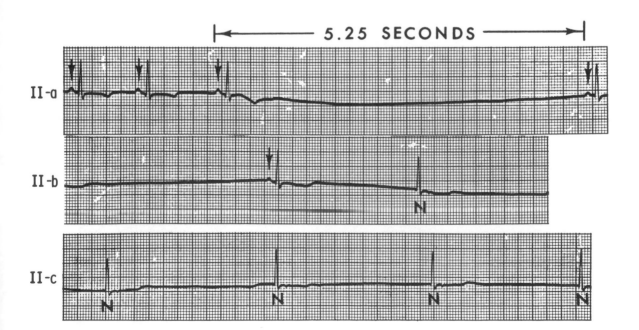

CASE 49: Diagnosis

The underlying cardiac rhythm is sinus (indicated by downward arrows), but there are episodes of sinus arrest (longest duration of sinus arrest: 5.25 seconds). Intermittently, AV junctional escape rhythm (marked N) occurs when the sinus node fails to produce sufficient cardiac impulses (sinus arrest).

It is interesting to note that the AV junctional escape rhythm is often slower than usual when there is significant dysfunction of the sinus node. The ventricular rate in AV junctional escape rhythm in this patient is only 25–27 beats/min (the usual rate ranging from 40 to 60 beats/min), indicating the diseased AV node.

These ECG findings represent far-advanced SSS (see Case 52) for which permanent artificial pacemaker implantation is urgently indicated. It has been shown that SSS often develops 10–15 years after successful surgical repair of atrial septal defect.

CASE 50

A 75-year-old man with a permanent artificial pacemaker was evaluated at the pacemaker clinic. He was not taking any medication, although he complained of palpitations.
1. What is the cardiac rhythm diagnosis?
2. What is the underlying cardiac disorder responsible for the production of this arrhythmia?
3. What is the proper therapeutic approach?

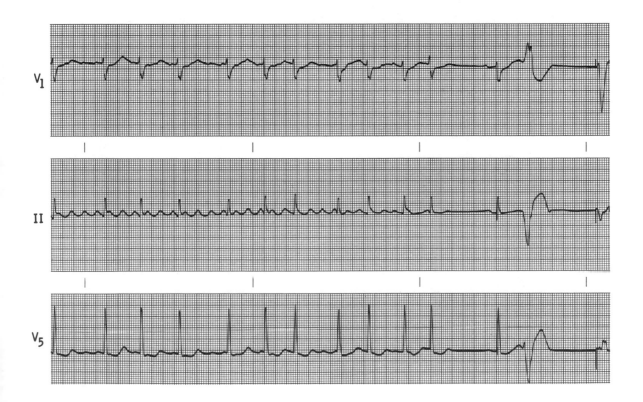

CASE 50: Diagnosis

His cardiac rhythms consist of atrial flutter—fibrillation, with only 1 sinus beat followed by a VPC and a demand pacemaker-induced ventricular beat. The artificial pacemaker activity is not present in most areas of this tracing simply because the ventricular rate during atrial flutter—fibrillation is faster than the preset pacing rate.

The underlying disorder responsible for the production of this arrhythmia is most likely SSS (see Case 52).

Antiarrhythmic drug therapy (e.g., quinidine) should be strongly considered if the cardiac rhythm is unstable and the patient is symptomatic (e.g., palpitations) for a long period of time even after permanent pacemaker implantation.

CASE 51

This ECG tracing was obtained from an elderly individual who complained of a near-syncope. The patient was not taking any medication.

1. What is the cardiac rhythm diagnosis?
2. What is the underlying disorder responsible for the production of this arrhythmia?
3. What is the proper therapeutic approach?

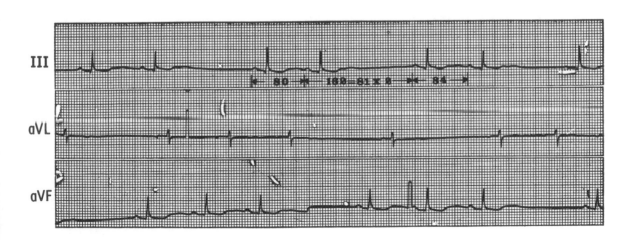

CASE 51: Diagnosis

The underlying cardiac rhythm is sinus, but there are many areas showing long P-P cycles. By a close observation, the long P-P interval is measured to be twice the basic P-P cycle. (The numbers represent hundredths of a second.) This ECG finding is termed "Mobitz type II SA block," which is manifested by intermittent 2:1 SA block in this tracing. Superficially, SA block simulates other arrhythmias, including sinus arrest, sinus bradycardia, and marked sinus arrhythmia.

It has been shown that SA block in one of the common manifestations of advanced SSS (see Case 52).

Permanent artificial pacemaker implantation is indicated.

CASE 52

A 46-year-old man was brought to the emergency room because he experienced several episodes of syncope or near-syncope. He was not taking any medication.
1. What is the cardiac rhythm diagnosis?
2. What is the underlying disorder responsible for the production of this arrhythmia?
3. What is the proper therapeutic approach?

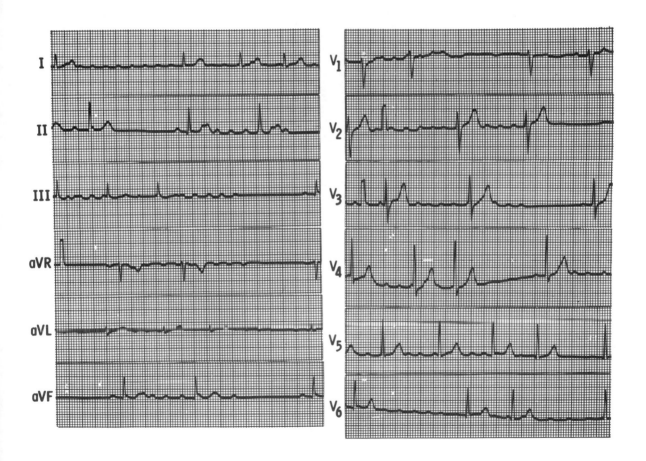

CASE 52: Diagnosis

The underlying cardiac rhythm is a very unstable sinus bradycardia, but atrial flutter with advanced AV block occurs intermittently. This ECG finding is the characteristic feature of advanced SSS.

Permanent artificial pacemaker implantation is definitely indicated.

Various ECG manifestation of SSS are summarized as follows:

Sick Sinus Syndrome: ECG Manifestations

1. Marked and persisting sinus bradycardia
2. Sinus arrest and/or SA block
3. Drug (e.g., atropine, isoproterenol)-resistant sinus bradyar-rhythmias
4. Long pause following an APC
5. Prolonged sinus node recovery time (more than 1500 msec) determined by atrial pacing
6. Chronic AF or repetitive occurrence of AF (less commonly atrial flutter):
   a. With slow ventricular rate
   b. Preceded or followed by sinus bradycardia, sinus arrest or SA block
7. AV junctional escape rhythm (with or without slow and unstable sinus activity)
8. Carotid sinus syncope (not every case)
9. Failure of restoration of sinus rhythm following cardioversion
10. Bradytachyarrhythmia syndrome
11. Common coexisting AV block and/or intraventricular block
12. Any combination of the above

CASE 53

A 66-year-old man was admitted to the intermediate CCU because he complained of slow pulse rate associated with dizziness and near-syncope. He was not taking any medication.
1. What is the cardiac rhythm diagnosis?
2. What is the underlying disorder responsible for the production of this arrhythmia?
3. What is the proper therapeutic approach?

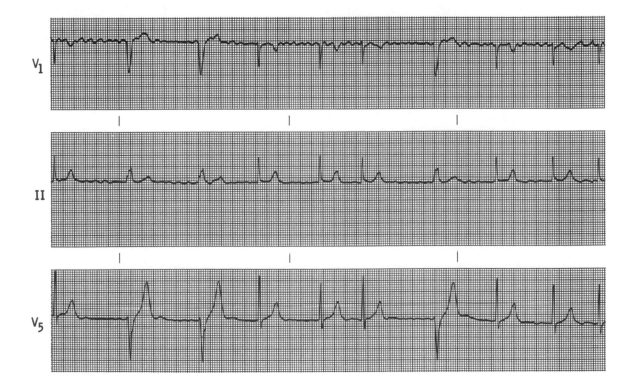

CASE 53: Diagnosis

The underlying cardiac rhythm is AF with advanced AV block, leading to intermittent ventricular escape (idioventricular) beats (the 2nd, 3rd, and 7th beats). This cardiac arrhythmia is, again, a manifestation of advanced SSS (see Case 52).

As far as the underlying reasons for the production of the ventricular escape beats in this ECG tracing are concerned, 2 major electrophysiologic events can be considered:

1. The site of AV block is within the AV node (AV nodal block), but the AV node is unable to produce the cardiac impulse as a result of the diseased AV node.
2. The site of AV block is distal to the AV node (infranodal block) so that ventricles produce the escape impulses.

At any rate, permanent artificial pacemaker implantation is definitely indicated.

Chapter 4
Atrial Arrhythmias

CASE 54

A 53-year-old man with CAD was examined at a cardiologist's office because he complained of palpitations. The only medication he had been taking was sublingual nitroglycerin as needed for angina.

1. What is the cardiac rhythm diagnosis?
2. Is there any other ECG abnormality?
3. What is the proper therapeutic approach to his arrhythmia?

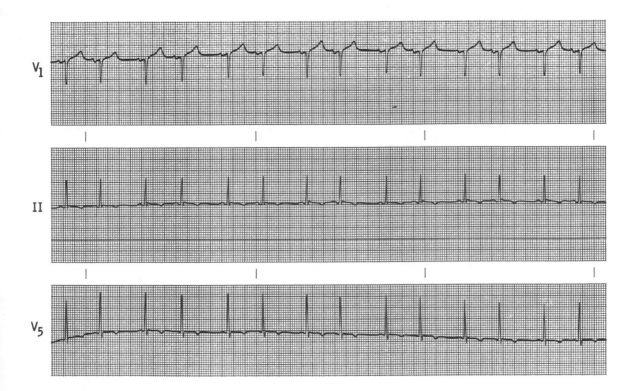

CASE 54: Diagnosis

The underlying cardiac rhythm is sinus (rate: 82 beats/min), but there are frequent APCs. Since the sinus beats appear alternatively with APCs, the diagnosis of atrial bigeminy is established.

Diffuse myocardial ischemia is also diagnosed on the basis of inverted T waves in leads II and V_5 and upright and tall T waves in lead V_1. (His 12-lead ECG reveals inverted T waves in practically all leads except for leads aVR and V_{1-2}—not shown here.)

By and large, no active treatment is necessary for APCs even if they occur frequently. However, symptomatic (for very sensitive individuals) APCs (e.g., palpitations) may require mild sedatives or small amounts of propranolol or quinidine. It is important to remember, however, that APCs or VPCs may often be induced by smoking or excessive consumption of coffee, tea, or cola drinks in some people. Thus, any causative factor should be eliminated if arrhythmia is thought to be induced by the above-mentioned items.

CASE 55

This ECG tracing was taken on a 73-year-old man with chronic CHF. He developed a new cardiac arrhythmia associated with worsening of his CHF in spite of maintenance digoxin therapy (0.25 mg daily by mouth).

1. What is the cardiac rhythm diagnosis?
·2. What is most likely the underlying cause of his arrhythmia?
3. What is the proper therapeutic approach?

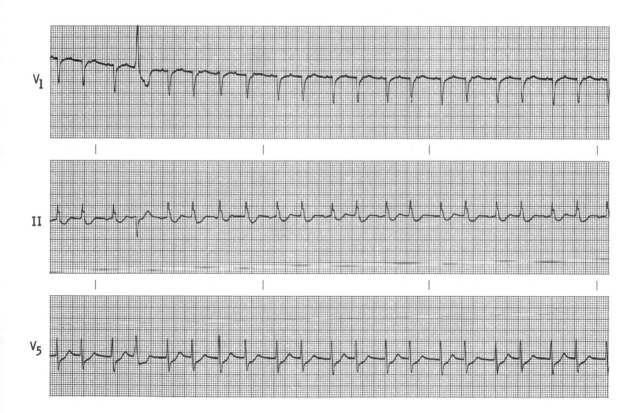

CASE 55: Diagnosis

At first glance, P waves are not clearly shown, and the ventricular cycle is irregular. However, rapidly appearing P waves are discernible by a close observation in leads V_1 and II. In addition, many readers should be able to recognize that the ventricular cycle has a regular irregularity (short and long R-R intervals alternate). Furthermore, the P-R intervals progressively lengthen until a blocked P wave occurs on every third P wave. Thus, the final rhythm diagnosis of this ECG tracing is atrial tachycardia (atrial rate: 180 beats/min) with 3:2 Wenckebach AV block. Atrial tachycardia with AV block (usually Wenckebach type) is often called "PAT with block."

As far as the underlying cause is concerned, atrial tachycardia with Wenckebach AV block is practically always a manifestation of digitalis intoxication, and immediate discontinuation of digitalis is the treatment of choice. When digitalis-induced arrhythmia is not immediately abolished following withdrawal of digitalis, potassium of phenytoin (Dilantin) may be indicated. Note a VPC (the 4th QRS complex).

CASE 56

This ECG tracing was taken on a 76-year-old man as a part of his annual medical checkup. He had no apparent complaint and was not taking any medication.

1. What is the cardiac rhythm diagnosis?

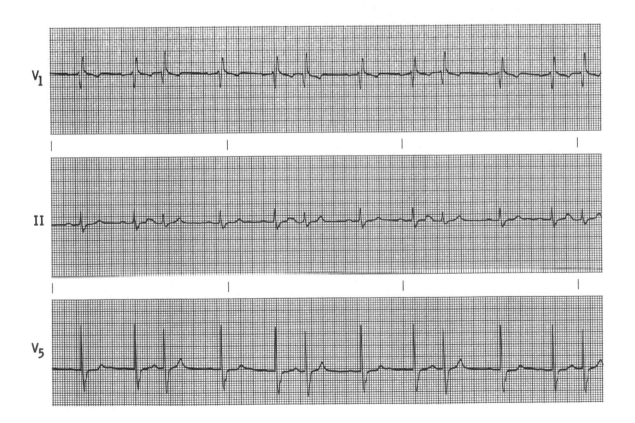

CASE 56: Diagnosis

The underlying cardiac rhythm is sinus (rate: 63 beats/min), but there are frequent APCs producing atrial trigeminy. The QRS complex of APCs is slightly different from that of the sinus beats because of slightly aberrant ventricular conduction. There is, of course, incomplete RBBB.

In general, no treatment is necessary for APCs as long as the patient is asymptomatic.

CASE 57

A 75-year old man was admitted to the CCU because a heart attack was diagnosed. He was not taking any drug before admission.
1. What is the cardiac rhythm diagnosis?
2. What is the ECG abnormality?
3. What is the proper therapeutic approach?

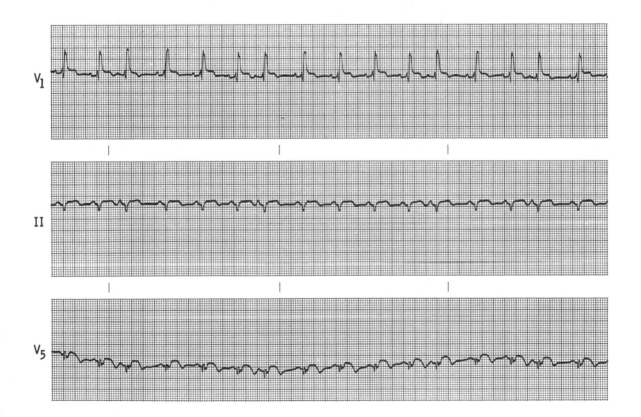

CASE 57: Diagnosis

The underlying cardiac rhythm is sinus (rate: 95 beats/min), but there are frequent APCs. The APCs in this ECG tracing are somewhat difficult to recognize simply because the underlying heart rate is relatively rapid.

His 12-lead ECG shows recent extensive anterior MI (except septum) as well as diaphragmatic (inferior) MI (only leads II and V_5 are shown here—Q or Q-S wave in these leads with S-T segment elevation with T wave inversion). In addition, the diagnosis of RBBB can be made without any difficulty.

No treatment is necessary for ABCs even in the presence of recent MI.

CASE 58

This ECG tracing was obtained from an 89-year-old man as a routine laboratory test. He has been relatively healthy for his age and was not taking any drug.
1. What is the cardiac rhythm diagnosis?
2. What is the proper therapeutic approach?

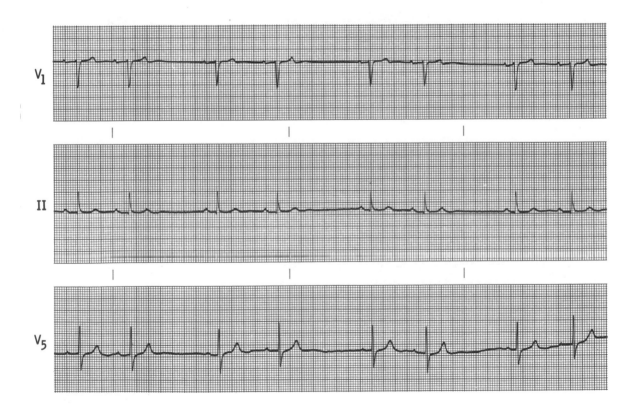

CASE 58: *Diagnosis*

The underlying cardiac rhythm is sinus (rate: 70 beats/min) with first degree AV block (P-R interval: 0.22 second). On superficial examination, 3:2 Wenckebach SA block (Mobitz type I SA block) can be diagnosed erroneously because the ventricular cycle exhibits a regular irregularity and the long R-R interval is shorter than the 2 basic R-R (or P-P) cycles. Otherwise, sinus arrhythmia or Wenckebach AV block may be diagnosed erroneously.

The correct diagnosis is frequent, blocked (nonconducted) APCs that occur on every third beat (blocked atrial trigeminy). The blocked ectopic P waves are best shown in lead V_1 by recognizing deformed T waves (the ectopic P wave is superimposed on the T wave). The blocked APCs occur when the premature atrial impulse is conducted while the AV node is absolutely refractory.

No treatment is necessary for blocked APCs.

CASE 59

This ECG tracing was taken on a 51-year-old woman because she complained of palpitations. She was not taking any medication.
1. What is the cardiac rhythm diagnosis?
2. What is the proper therapeutic approach?

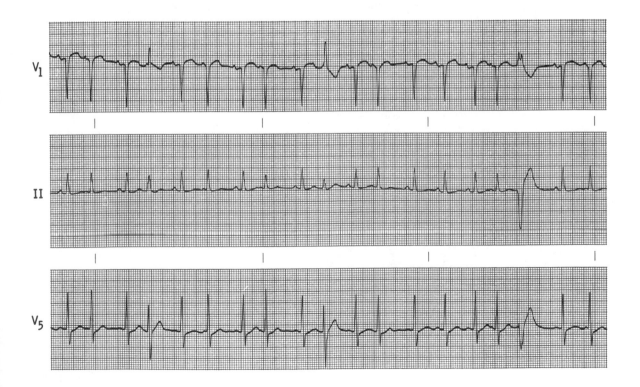

V₁

II

V₅

CASE 59: Diagnosis

The underlying cardiac rhythm is sinus tachycardia (rate: 108 beats/min), but there are frequent APCs. It should be noted that there are several different kinds of ectopic P waves and the coupling intervals also vary. Therefore, multifocal APCs can be diagnosed. In addition, some APCs are followed by bizarre QRS complexes (the 4th and 10th beats) as a result of aberrant ventricular conduction. There is a VPC (the 17th beat).

Multifocal APCs may lead to multifocal atrial tachycardia, but no active treatment is necessary for APCs alone, even multifocal in origin, as long as the patient is asymptomatic. However, small amounts of quinidine or propranolol may be used if the APCs produce significant symptoms (e.g., palpitations). Any possible etiologic factor (e.g., excessive consumption of coffee or tea) should be eliminated.

CASE 60

A 76-year-old man was examined at the cardiac clinic at a periodic medical checkup. He had no complaint and was not taking any medication.
1. What is the cardiac rhythm diagnosis?

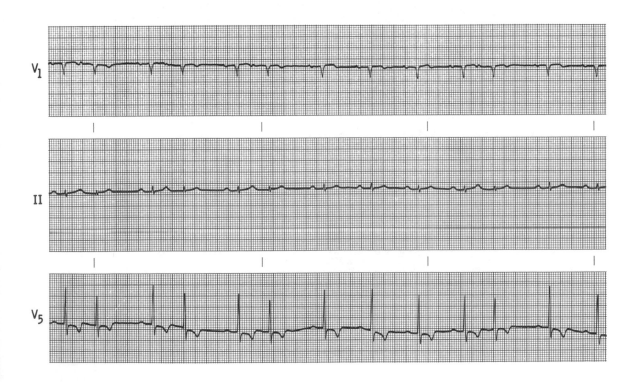

CASE 60: Diagnosis

The underlying cardiac rhythm is sinus (rate: 71 beats/min) with first degree AV block (P-R interval: 0.22 second). There are frequent APCs, producing an area of atrial bigeminy (the first half of the tracing).

Note that the P-R interval of the APC is markedly prolonged in this tracing for 2 major reasons. First, the ectopic P wave occurs very early (short coupling interval) so that the AV node is extremely refractory (almost its absolute refractory period) when the ectopic atrial impulse is conducted. Second, there is the preexisting AV conduction disturbance (first degree AV block during sinus rhythm). In addition, the QRS complexes of the APCs show slight aberrant ventricular conduction.

Lateral myocardial ischemia is considered (inverted T wave in lead V_5).

CASE 61

A 76-year-old woman with mild hypertension was seen at the hypertensive clinic at a routine visit. She had been taking hydrochlorothiazide 50 mg every other day by mouth for several years. She had no complaint.

1. What is the cardiac rhythm diagnosis?

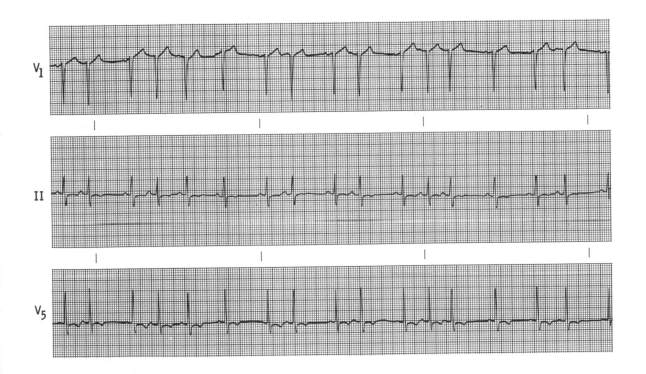

CASE 61: Diagnosis

The underlying cardiac rhythm is sinus (rate: 78 beats/min), but there are frequent APCs. The term "atrial group beats" is used when APCs occur consecutively up to 5 beats in a row. When 6 or more APCs occur consecutively, the term "atrial tachycardia" is used (see Case 66).

No active treatment is necessary for APCs even when they occur as atrial group beats. Atrial group beats often lead to atrial tachycardia (see Case 66).

CASE 62

This ECG tracing was obtained from a 49-year-old man with cardiomyopathy. He had no particular complaint and was not taking any drug.
1. What is the cardiac rhythm diagnosis?
2. What is the proper therapeutic approach?

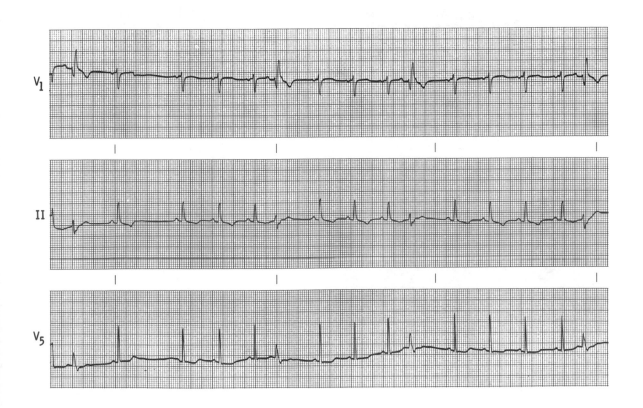

CASE 62: Diagnosis

The underlying cardiac rhythm is sinus (rate: 90 beats/min), but there are frequent APCs. All APCs are followed by bizarre QRS complexes as a result of aberrant ventricular conduction. Aberrant ventricular conduction occurs when the atrial premature impulse is conducted to the ventricles during their partial refractory period.

In addition, there is a blocked (nonconducted) APC (the 2nd APC) following a postectopic pause. This particular APC is blocked as a result of Ashman's phenomenon, that is, the AV junction is absolutely refractory under this circumstance following a long postectopic pause because the refractoriness of the heart (including AV junction) is directly influenced by the preceding cardiac cycle. In other words, the longer the ventricular cycle (R-R interval) the longer is the refractory period following it; the shorter the ventricular cycle the shorter is the refractory period.

No active treatment is necessary for APCs.

CASE 63

A 62-year-old man with a previous history of diaphragmatic MI was seen at the cardiac clinic at a follow-up visit. He was free of any cardiac symptoms and not taking any drug.
1. What is the cardiac rhythm diagnosis?
2. What is the proper therapeutic approach?

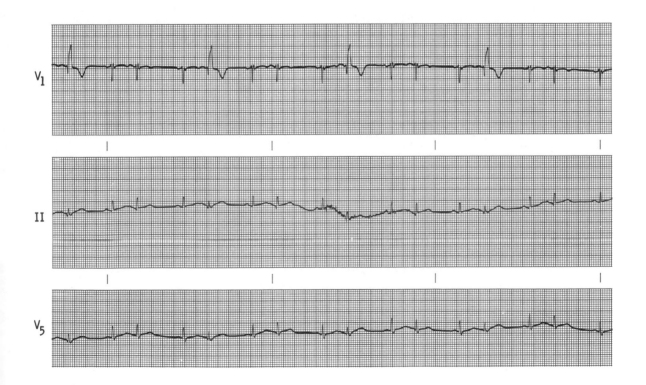

CASE 63: Diagnosis

The underlying cardiac rhythm is sinus with a rate of 90 beats/min. There are frequent APCs producing atrial bigeminy, and every other APC demonstrates aberrant ventricular conduction. Aberrant ventricular conduction occurs when the premature atrial impulse is conducted to the ventricles during their partial refractory period. However, the exact reason that every other APC shows aberrant ventricular conduction is not clear. Obviously, APCs with aberrant ventricular conduction closely mimic VPCs, but bizarre QRS complexes preceded by the premature P waves exclude the possibility of VPCs.

No treatment is needed for APCs.

CASE 64

Cardiac consultation was requested on an 82-year-old woman for evaluation of her arrhythmia. She was not taking any medication and was free of any cardiac symptoms.
1. What is the cardiac rhythm diagnosis?
2. What is the proper therapeutic approach?

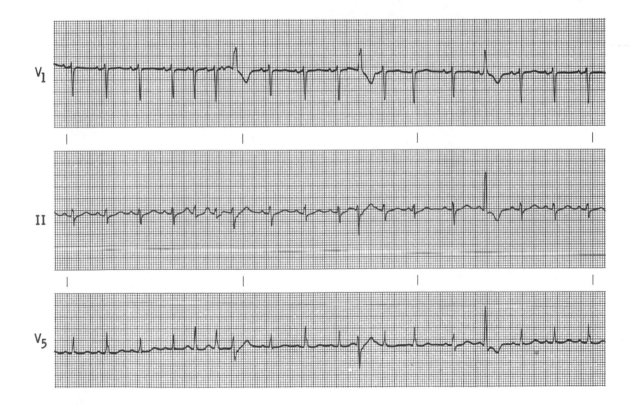

CASE 64: Diagnosis

The underlying cardiac rhythm is sinus tachycardia with a rate of 105 beats/min. There are frequent multifocal APCs with atrial group beats (up to 3 beats in a row), and some of them are followed by aberrant ventricular conduction. APCs with aberrant ventricular conduction superficially resemble VPCs. Note a VPC with a fusion beat (the 15th beat).

No active treatment is necessary for APCs, even with group beats, as long as the patient is asymptomatic.

CASE 65

A 52-year-old woman was brought to the emergency room because she developed palpitations suddenly. She had no prior history of known heart disease and was not taking any medication.
1. What is the cardiac rhythm diagnosis?
2. What is the proper therapeutic approach?

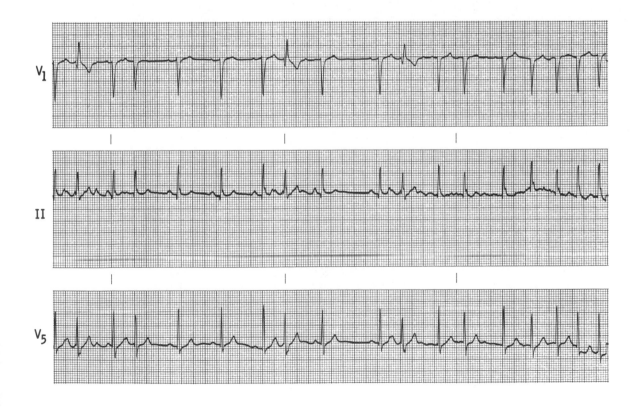

CASE 65: Diagnosis

The underlying cardiac rhythm is sinus with a rate of 82 beats/min. There are frequent APCs with aberrant ventricular conduction leading to intermittent paroxysmal atrial flutter–fibrillation. It is a well-known fact that any type of atrial tachyarrhythmias is often initiated by frequent APCs.

Possible underlying causes (e.g., stress, anxiety, smoking, excessive consumption of coffee) of the development of this arrhythmia should be eliminated if present. Otherwise, small amounts of quinidine may be given by mouth to suppress this atrial arrhythmia.

A possibility of SSS should be considered always when dealing with recurrent AF or atrial flutter, especially in elderly people.

CASE 66

This ECG tracing was obtained from a 59-year-old man who complained of an "unpleasant feeling in the chest," which seemed to occur during stressful situations. He was not taking any medication.
1. What is the cardiac rhythm diagnosis?
2. What is the proper therapeutic approach?

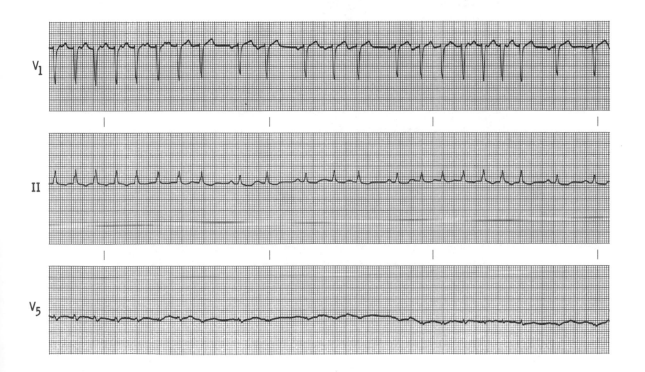

CASE 66: *Diagnosis*

The underlying cardiac rhythm is sinus with a rate of 90 beats/min. Paroxysmal atrial tachycardia (rate: 170 beats/min) is initiated by frequent APCs.

Any stressful factors that may cause this arrhythmia should be eliminated if possible. If this atrial arrhythmia recurs, propranolol will be the drug of choice under this circumstance. It has been well documented that beta-blockers are extremely effective for various tachyarrhythmias induced by anxiety, emotional upset, and a variety of stress factors.

CASE 67

Cardiac consultation was requested because a 30-year-old woman suddenly developed a rapid heart action. There was no prior history of known heart disease, but she had had similar episodes in the past. She was not taking any medication.

1. What is the cardiac rhythm diagnosis?
2. What is the proper therapeutic approach?

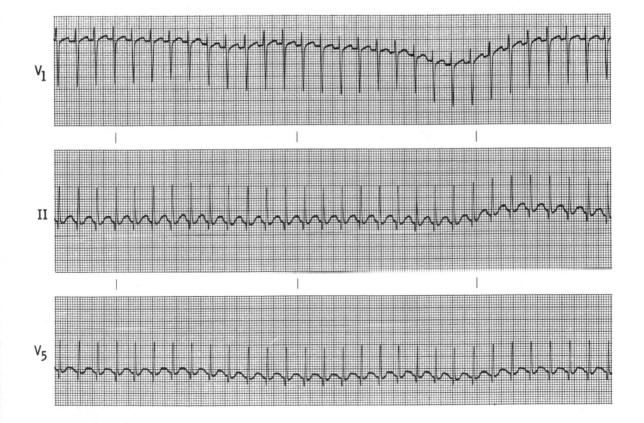

CASE 67: Diagnosis

The cardiac rhythm is supraventricular tachycardia (most likely atrial tachycardia) with a rate of 198 beats/min. The cardiac cycle is regular, and the QRS complexes are normal. The P waves are not clearly discernible because of their superimposition to the T waves of the preceding beats.

When dealing with supreventricular tachycardia, the first therapeutic approach is to apply carotid sinus stimulation (CSS). CSS is often effective in terminating supraventricular tachycardia. If CSS is found to be ineffective, propranolol should be tried next. Digitalis or verapamil will be the next drug of choice. When CSS and the above-mentioned drugs are ineffective, an electrophysiologic study should be considered.

There are 3 major possibilities of underlying causes of supraventricular tachycardia: hyperthyroidism, mitral valve prolapse syndrome (MVPS), and Wolff-Parkinson-White (WPW) syndrome. These disorders should be investigated whenever any patient develops supraventricular tachyarrhythmias for unknown reasons.

CASE 68

This ECG tracing was obtained from an 82-year-old woman. She was not taking any medication.
1. What is the cardiac rhythm diagnosis?
2. What is most likely the underlying disorder?
3. What is the proper therapeutic approach?

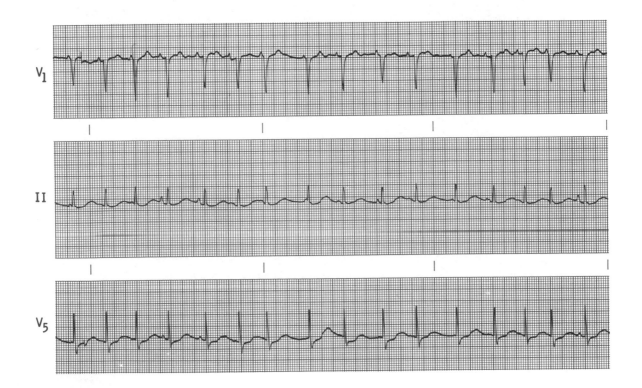

V₁

II

V₅

CASE 68: Diagnosis

The cardiac rhythm is multifocal atrial tachycardia (MAT) with a rate of 100 beats/min. It should be noted that the P wave configuration and the P-P cycle vary throughout. In addition, the P-R intervals also vary. These findings are characteristic features of MAT. There are also, frequent AV junctional (slightly accelerated) escape beats (the 8th, 10th and 12th QRS complexes). The atrial rate in MAT may be as rapid as 160–250 beats/min, but more commonly the rate is relatively slower (100–140 beats/min) than the ordinary paroxysmal atrial tachycardia.

As the underlying disorder, COPD is the most common disease associated with MAT. Thus, the proper treatment of the underlying pulmonary disease is the more important and more effective therapeutic approach to MAT. The efficacy of commonly used antiarrhythmic agents are often disappointing in the treatment of MAT.

CASE 69

A 77-year-old woman with a long-standing pulmonary emphysema was brought to the emergency room because of a rapid heart action. She was not taking any medication.
1. What is the cardiac rhythm diagnosis?
2. What is the proper therapeutic approach?

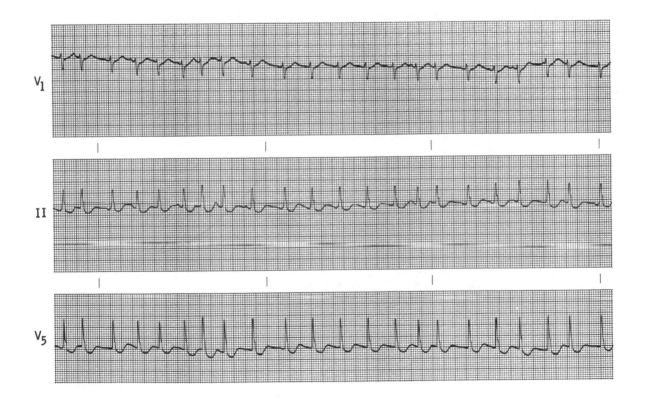

V₁

II

V₅

CASE 69: Diagnosis

On superficial examination, the cardiac rhythm appears to be AF because the cardiac cycle is irregular and no P waves are clearly evident. However, the correct diagnosis of this ECG tracing is again MAT with rapid ventricular response (rate: 120–150 beats/min). By a close observation, the P waves with many different types can be appreciated, and the P-P cycles vary.

Aggressive treatment of the underlying pulmonary disease is the most effective therapeutic approach to MAT. Digitalis and antiarrhythmic agents (e.g., quinidine) may be tried with caution, but the therapeutic result is often not favorable as long as the underlying pulmonary disease is not well managed.

CASE 70

A 69-year-old woman was examined at the general medical clinic at a periodic checkup.
1. What is the cardiac rhythm diagnosis?

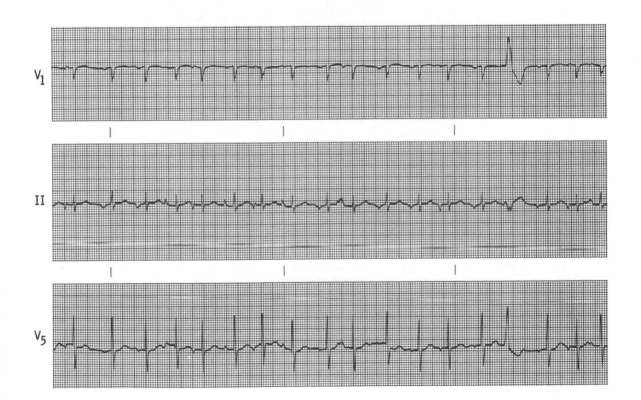

CASE 70: Diagnosis

This ECG finding is another good example of MAT. Note that there are many kinds of P waves, and the P-P cycles as well as the P-R intervals vary. In contrast to the ECG findings shown in Cases 68 and 69, many P waves are inverted in lead II but different in degree. Note a VPC (the 15th beat).

Again, the patient was found to have advanced COPD. It should be recognized that many P waves demonstrate a tent-shaped sharp tip (either upright or inverted in lead II).

CASE 71

A 73-year-old woman with known COPD was examined at the pulmonary clinic.
1. What is the cardiac rhythm diagnosis?
2. What is the proper therapeutic approach?

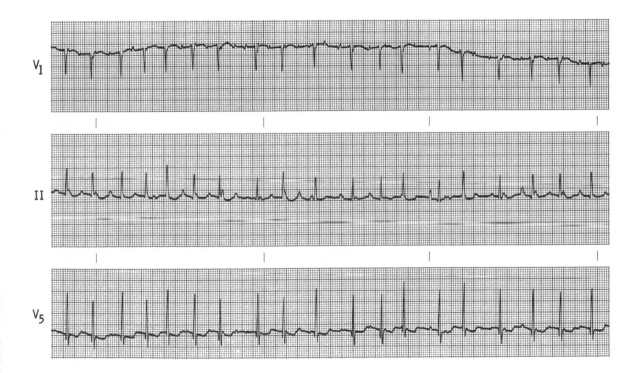

CASE 71: Diagnosis

At glance, the cardiac rhythm appears to be AF or atrial flutter because the ventricular cycle is grossly irregular and the atrial activities seem to be chaotic. The correct diagnosis is, however, MAT with varying AV block. In this tracing, the atrial rate of MAT ranges from 200 to 250 beats/min, and this finding is in contrast to the relatively slow atrial rate in Cases 68, 69, and 70. Note that many P waves are not conducted to the ventricles.

Again, the best therapeutic approach to MAT is proper treatment of the underlying pulmonary disease. If MAT with rapid ventricular rate persists, digitalis and antiarrhythmic agents (e.g., quinidine)may be tried with caution.

CASE 72

This ECG tracing was obtained from a 79-year-old man with previous history of anterior MI associated with COPD. He was not taking any medication.
1. What is the cardiac rhythm diagnosis?
2. What is the proper therapeutic approach?

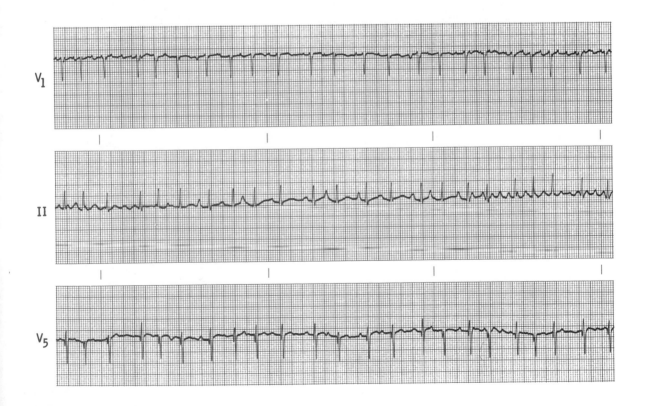

V1

II

V5

CASE 72: *Diagnosis*

The underlying cardiac rhythm is multifocal atrial tachycardia (rate: 120–140 beats/min), but paroxysmal atrial flutter–fibrillation occurs intermittently (at the beginning and the end of the tracing). Many P waves are peaked and tall (P-pulmonale) because of the underlying COPD.

First, his pulmonary function should be improved for the cardiac arrhythmia. When MAT with intermittent atrial flutter–fibrillation persists or recurs even after proper treatment of his pulmonary disease, digitalization with or without antiarrhythmic drug therapy (e.g., quinidine) may be carried out with caution. The efficacy of digitalis and various antiarrhythmic drugs is often disappointing for MAT.

CASE 73

A 59-year-old woman was admitted to the CCU because of chest pain of 2–3 hours' duration associated with rapid heart action. She was not taking any drug.
1. What is the cardiac rhythm diagnosis?
2. What is the ECG diagnosis?
3. What is the proper therapeutic approach?

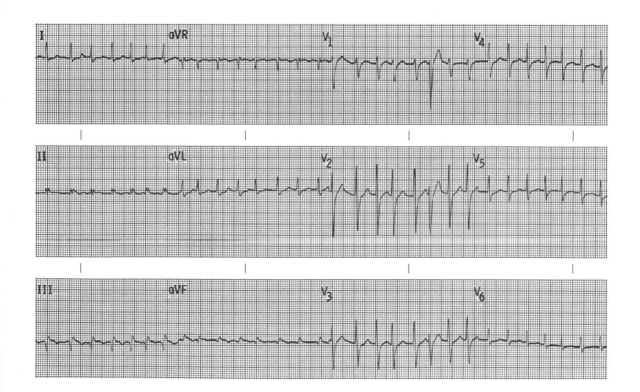

CASE 73: *Diagnosis*

The cardiac rhythm is AF with rapid ventricular response (rate: 150–200 beats/min) and occasional VPCs. The diagnosis of acute diaphragmatic MI can be made on the basis of abnormal Q waves in leads III and aVF associated with S-T segment elevation.

The treatment of choice for AF with rapid ventricular response is rapid digitalization even in the presence of acute MI. However, a smaller than usual dosage should be used for patients with acute MI. If the clinical situation is extremely urgent, immediate application of DC shock is the treatment of choice.

CASE 74

This ECG tracing was obtained from a 73-year-old man with recent heart attack. He was not taking any medication.
1. What is the cardiac rhythm diagnosis?
2. What is the ECG diagnosis?
3. What is the proper therapeutic approach?

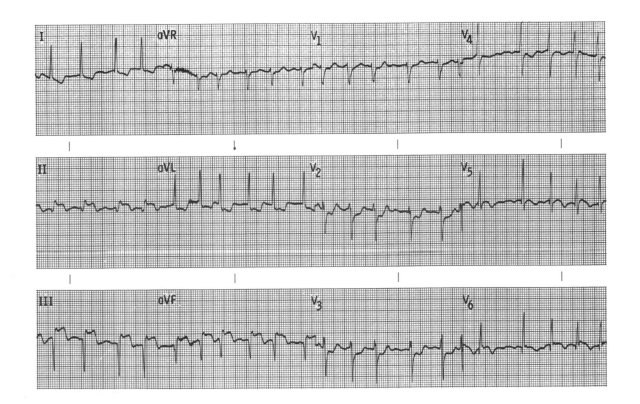

CASE 74: Diagnosis

The cardiac rhythm is AF with moderately rapid ventricular response (rate: 105–125 beats/min). Recent diaphragmatic MI is diagnosed without any difficulty. In addition, posterolateral myocardial ischemia is considered. S-T segment depression in leads V_{1-3} is most likely due to posterior subepicardial injury. Left ventricular hypertrophy is also diagnosed.

Moderately rapid digitalization is the treatment of choice.

CASE 75

A 73-year-old man with CAD was seen at the cardiac clinic 3 weeks after discharge from the hospital. He had no particular complaint and was not taking any drug.
1. What is the cardiac rhythm diagnosis?
2. What is the proper therapeutic approach?

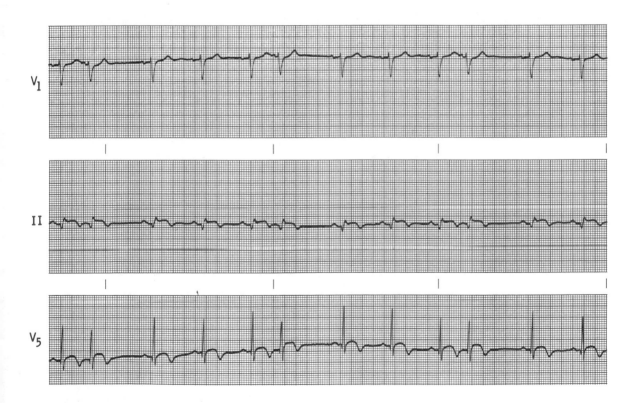

CASE 75: Diagnosis

The underlying cardiac rhythm is sinus with a rate of 68 beats/min. There are frequent APCs producing atrial quadrigeminy. The QRS complexes following APCs demonstrate a slightly bizarre configuration because of aberrant ventricular conduction.

No treatment is necessary for APCs even in the presence of recent diaphragmatic MI (5 weeks old).

CASE 76

A 61-year-old woman with mild hypertension was brought to the emergency room because of rapid heart action. She was not taking any medication.
1. What is the cardiac rhythm diagnosis?
2. What is the proper therapeutic approach?

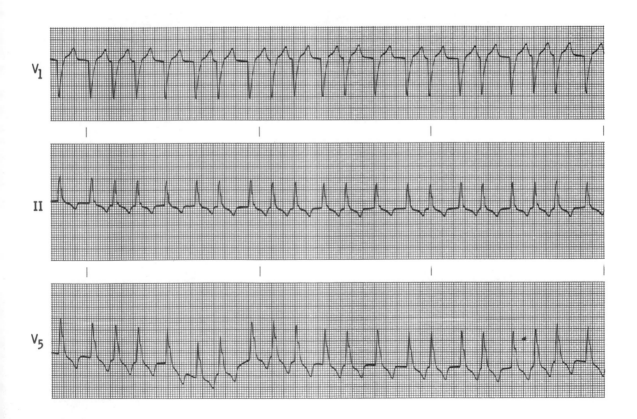

CASE 76: Diagnosis

The cardiac rhythm is AF with rapid ventricular response (rate: 130–145 beats/min). The QRS complexes are broad and bizarre because of the preexisting LBBB. Ventricular tachycardia is superficially simulated, but a grossly irregular ventricular cycle excludes such possibility.

The treatment of choice is rapid or moderately rapid digitalization.

CASE 77

A 59-year-old man was admitted to the intermediate CCU because of acute CHF associated with rapid heart action. He was not taking any medication on admission.
1. What is the cardiac rhythm diagnosis?
2. What is the proper therapeutic approach?

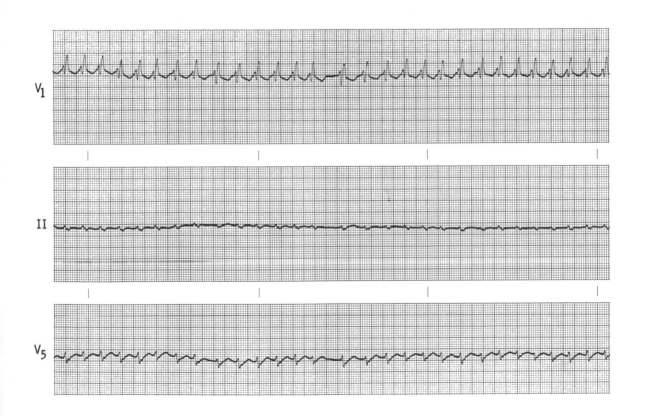

V₁

II

V₅

CASE 77: Diagnosis

The cardiac rhythm is AF with rapid ventricular response (rate: 175 beats/min). The QRS complexes are slightly bizarre and broad because of incomplete RBBB. Again, ventricular tachycardia is superficially simulated.

The treatment of choice is rapid digitalization. If the clinical situation is extremely urgent, immediate application of direct current (DC) shock is the treatment of choice.

CASE 78

This ECG tracing was taken on a 73-year-old woman. She was brought to the emergency room because of palpitations with acute onset. She was not taking any medication.

1. What is the cardiac rhythm diagnosis?
2. What is the proper therapeutic approach?

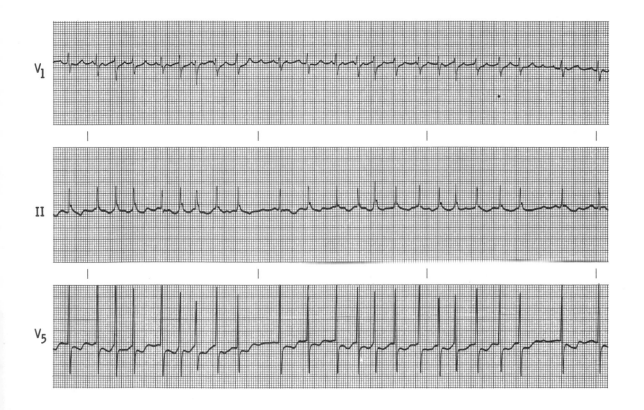

V₁

II

V₅

CASE 78: Diagnosis

The cardiac rhythm is atrial flutter–fibrillation with rapid ventricular response (rate: 140–180 beats/min). Some QRS complexes are slightly deformed as a result of slightly aberrant ventricular conduction.

The term "atrial flutter–fibrillation" is used when the cardiac rhythm is a mixed form between atrial flutter and AF.

The treatment of choice is rapid digitalization. If the clinical situation is extremely urgent, however, immediate application of DC shock is the treatment of choice.

Left ventricular hypertrophy is considered.

CASE 79

Cardiac consultation was requested on a 74-year-old man with known CAD (history of diaphragmatic MI 2 years previously) for evaluation of his cardiac arrhythmia. He was not taking any medication and was asymptomatic.

1. What is the cardiac rhythm diagnosis?
2. What is the proper therapeutic approach?

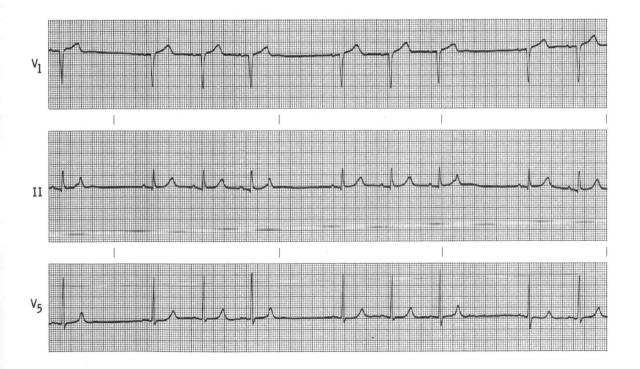

CASE 79: Diagnosis

The underlying cardiac rhythm is sinus with a rate of 68 beats/min. By superficial examination, the cardiac rhythm appears to be Wenckebach SA block (4:3 conduction). Otherwise, the rhythm may be misdiagnosed as marked sinus arrhythmia or intermittent sinus arrest.

The correct diagnosis, however, is frequent, blocked (nonconducted) APCs producing blocked atrial quadrigeminy. It should be noted that the premature P wave (blocked APC) is superimposed on the top of the T wave of the preceding beat so that the T wave is markedly deformed.

No treatment is necessary for blocked APCs.

CASE 80

A 72-year-old man was evaluated at a cardiologist's office because he experienced several episodes of near-syncope and dizziness. He was not taking any medication.
1. What is the cardiac rhythm diagnosis?
2. What is most likely the underlying disorder?
3. What is the proper therapeutic approach?

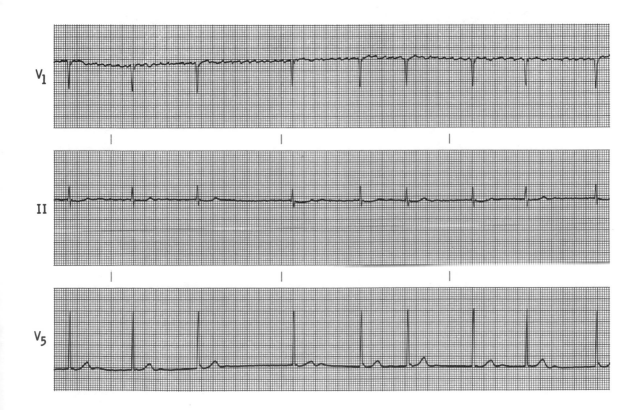

CASE 80: *Diagnosis*

The underlying cardiac rhythm is AF, but the ventricular rate is very slow (rate: 43–50 beats/min). In addition, some R-R intervals are regular. Therefore, the complete rhythm diagnosis of this ECG tracing is AF with advanced AV block causing intermittent AV junctional escape beats.

As far as the underlying disorder responsible for production of this arrhythmia is concerned, advanced SSS is the most likely possibility. Permanent artificial pacing is recommended for symptomatic or advanced SSS (see Case 52). The Holter monitor ECG is highly recommended to document his arrhythmia correlated with his symptoms (e.g., near-syncope).

CASE 81

A 61-year-old man with mild hypertension was seen in the emergency room because of rapid heart action. He was not taking any medication.
1. What is the cardiac rhythm diagnosis?
2. What is the proper therapeutic approach?

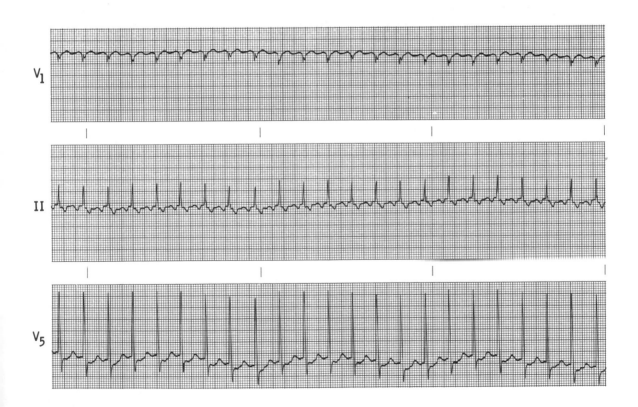

CASE 81: Diagnosis

The cardiac rhythm is atrial flutter (atrial rate: 282 beats/min) with 2:1 AV conduction (ventricular rate: 141 beats/min). Note that the ventricular cycle is precisely regular, and every other atrial flutter wave is conducted to the ventricles. Under this circumstance, "2:1 AV conduction" is a correct expression rather than "2:1 AV block" simply because it is a physiologic phenomenon.

To anyone not familiar with atrial flutter with 2:1 AV conduction, the arrhythmia may be misdiagnosed as supraventricular tachycardia (SVT) or even sinus tachycardia. When dealing with a regular rapid tachycardia (rate: around 150 beats/min) with normal QRS complexes, a possibility of atrial flutter with 2:1 AV conduction should always be considered, especially when the usual P waves are not discernible.

Rapid digitalization is the treatment of choice under this circumstance. If the clinical situation is extremely urgent (e.g., hypotension as a result of rapid heart rate), immediate application of DC shock is the treatment of choice. In general, DC shock (usually with a low energy setting) is very effective to terminate atrial flutter.

Left ventricular hypertrophy is considered.

CASE 82

A 79-year-old man was evaluated at the medical service because of his cardiac arrhythmia. He was not taking any medication.
1. What is the cardiac rhythm diagnosis?
2. What is the proper therapeutic approach?

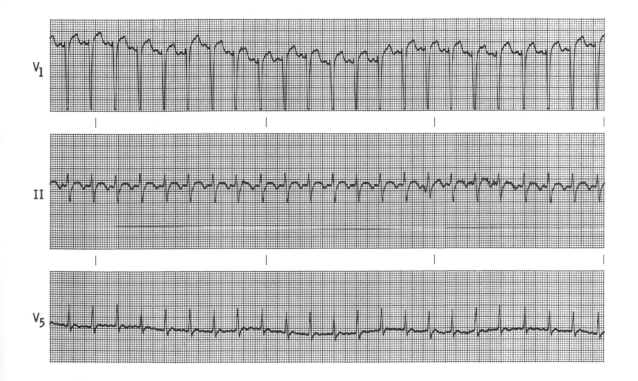

CASE 82: Diagnosis

The cardiac rhythm is atrial flutter (atrial rate: 286 beats/min) with 2:1 AV conduction (ventricular rate: 143 beats/min). Note that the ventricular cycle is precisely regular, and every other atrial flutter wave is conducted to the ventricles. Every other atrial flutter wave is not clearly evident because of superimposition to the end portion of the QRS complexes.

The diagnostic features and the therapeutic approach to atrial flutter with 2:1 AV conduction have been described in detail in Case 81.

Left anterior hemiblock is strongly considered.

CASE 83

A 58-year-old woman was presented at the weekly cardiology conference because her cardiac arrhythmia was considered to be somewhat unusual. She was taking a cardiac drug for her arrhythmia.
1. What is the cardiac rhythm diagnosis?
2. What cardiac drug was this patient most likely taking?
3. What is the proper therapeutic approach?

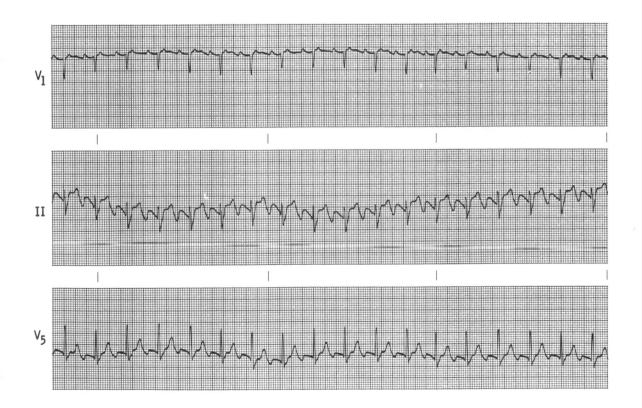

CASE 83: *Diagnosis*

At first glance, large inverted P waves seem to be present before each QRS complex, and the R-R intervals are regular with normal QRS complexes. Thus, inexperienced readers may misdiagnose this rhythm as AV junctional tachycardia. Otherwise, it may be diagnosed erroneously as supraventricular tachycardia, atrial tachycardia, or even sinus tachycardia.

The correct diagnosis, however, is atrial flutter (atrial rate: 216 beats/min) with 2:1 AV response (ventricular rate: 108/min). The atrial flutter waves are best shown in lead V_1. The atrial rate in this atrial flutter is slower than usual (the usual atrial flutter cycle ranging from 250 to 350 beats/min) because of the quinidine effect.

This patient was given quinidine 0.3 g 4 times daily by mouth to terminate the atrial flutter. It should be noted, however, that quinidine should not be given alone under this circumstance because quinidine causes slowing of atrial rate and enhancement of AV conduction, leading to atrial flutter with 1:1 AV conduction. When this occurs, the ventricular rate will be increased because of 1:1 AV conduction even though the atrial flutter cycle becomes slower. Therefore, digitalization must be carried out first when dealing with atrial flutter with 2:1 AV conduction. Digitalis alone is often successful in terminating atrial flutter. Quinidine may be added later if necessary when the sinus rhythm is not restored with digitalis alone.

CASE 84

This ECG tracing was obtained from a 59-year-old man with advanced CHF. He was given several medications, including digitalis, quinidine, and diuretics.
1. What is the cardiac rhythm diagnosis?
2. What is the proper therapeutic approach?

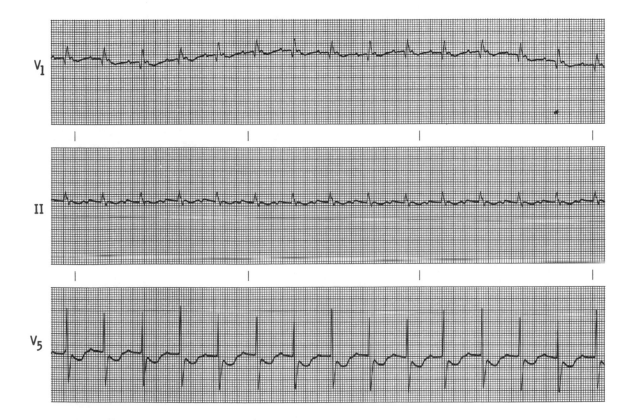

CASE 84: Diagnosis

The cardiac rhythm is atrial flutter (atrial rate: 184 beats/min) with 2:1 AV conduction. The atrial flutter waves are clearly evident in lead V_1. The diagnosis of incomplete RBBB can be established without any difficulty.

The atrial flutter cycle is much slower than usual (the usual flutter cycle: 250–350 beats/min) because of the quinidine effect. Again, atrial flutter with 2:1 AV conduction should be treated with digitalis first. In many cases, digitalis alone is effective in terminating atrial flutter with 2:1 AV conduction. Thus, quinidine is not necessary once sinus rhythm is restored with digitalis alone. When atrial flutter persists even after full digitalization, quinidine may be added later in order to terminate atrial flutter. DC shock should be applied immediately when the clinical situation is extremely urgent in patients with atrial flutter with 2:1 AV conduction. DC shock is found to be very effective in terminating atrial flutter.

CASE 85

A 73-year-old woman was brought to the emergency room because of rapid heart action. She was not taking any medication.
1. What is the cardiac rhythm diagnosis?
2. What is the proper therapeutic approach?

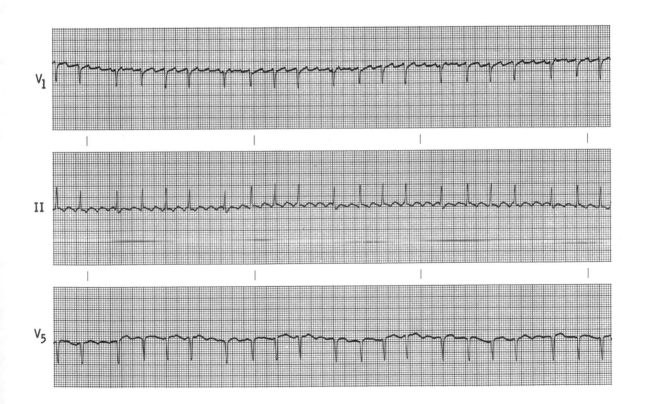

CASE 85: Diagnosis

The cardiac rhythm is atrial flutter (atrial rate: 300 beats/min) with Wenckebach AV response. Note that 4 ventricular group beats are followed by a ventricular pause, leading to a regular irregularity of the ventricular cycle. The long ventricular pause is shorter than 2 short ventricular cycles—the characteristic feature of the Wenckebach AV conduction.

The treatment of choice is digitalization (rapid or moderately rapid method).

CASE 86

This ECG tracing was obtained a few hours later on a 73-year-old woman (the same patient shown in Case 85) following digitalization.
1. What is the cardiac rhythm diagnosis?

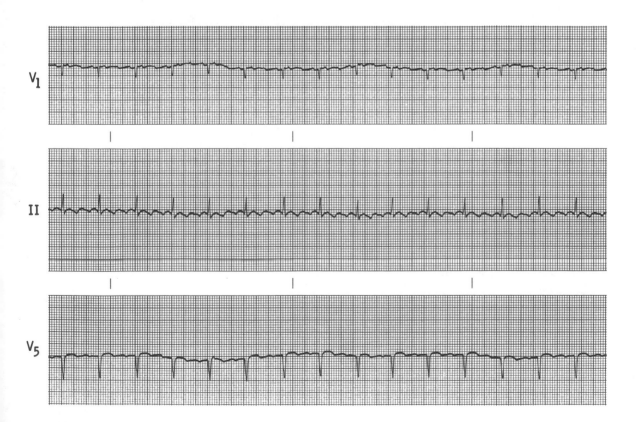

V₁

II

V₅

CASE 86: Diagnosis

The cardiac rhythm is atrial flutter (atrial rate: 300 beats/min) with 3:1 AV block (ventricular rate: 100 beats/min). The ventricular cycle is precisely regular in this tracing because the AV conduction ratios (3:1 AV block) remain constant. The conduction ratios showing odd numbers (e.g., 3:1 or 5:1) in atrial flutter are very rare. In most untreated cases, atrial flutter reveals 2:1 AV conduction. Atrial flutter with 1:1 AV conduction is extremely unusual.

CASE 87

A 68-year-old man with a previous history of MI was seen at the cardiac clinic at a periodic checkup. He had been taking digoxin 0.25 mg daily by mouth.

1. What is the cardiac rhythm diagnosis?
2. What is the proper therapeutic approach?

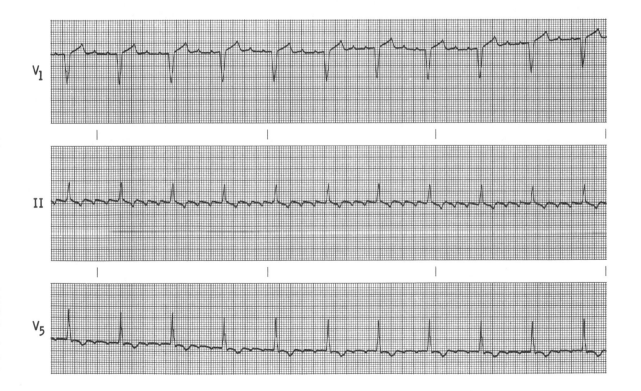

CASE 87: *Diagnosis*

The cardiac rhythm is atrial flutter (atrial rate: 268 beats/min) with 4:1 AV block. Note that every 4th atrial flutter wave is conducted to the ventricles so that the ventricular cycle is precisely regular (ventricular rate: 67 beats/min).

In atrial flutter, 4:1 AV block is usually not a manifestation of digitalis toxicity. If atrial flutter has been present for many years (more than 5 years), a possibility of a restoration of sinus rhythm is extremely remote. Therefore, one should not attempt to terminate atrial flutter by any antiarrhythmic agent (e.g., quinidine) or DC shock. In fact, DC shock should be avoided under this circumstance because the procedure may provoke more serious arrhythmias when a patient is taking digitalis (any amount). In addition, the underlying disorder responsible for the production of chronic atrial flutter or fibrillation is often advanced SSS (see Case 52). Thus, in either case, DC shock is extremely hazardous.

CASE 88

A 71-year-old man with chronic CHF associated with mild hypertension was examined at the medical clinic. He has been taking digoxin 0.25 mg and hydrochlorothiazide 25 mg daily by mouth.
1. What is the cardiac rhythm diagnosis?
2. What ECG abnormality is present?

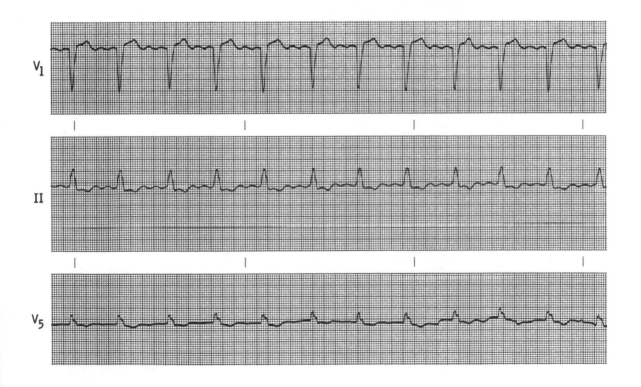

CASE 88: Diagnosis

At first glance, the atrial activity is not evident, and the ventricular cycle is regular with broad QRS complexes. The correct cardiac rhythm diagnosis is atrial flutter (atrial rate: 288 beats/min) with 4:1 AV block because every 4th atrial flutter wave is conducted to the ventricles. The atrial flutter waves are discernible in lead V_1 (not as clear as other ECG tracings, such as in Case 87). The diagnosis of LBBB can be entertained without any difficulty.

The proper therapeutic approach has been described in Case 87.

CASE 89

This ECG tracing of a 70-year-old woman was presented to the weekly ECG conference because her arrhythmia was thought to be somewhat unusual.
1. What is the cardiac rhythm diagnosis?

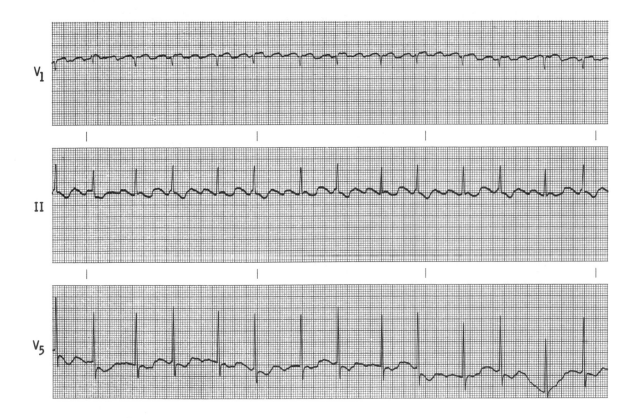

V_1

II

V_5

CASE 89: Diagnosis

It is obvious that the ventricular cycle shows a regular irregularity. In other words, short and long R-R intervals alternate throughout the tracing. By close observation, most readers should see that the long R-R interval is shorter than 3 atrial flutter cycles, whereas the short R-R interval is longer than 2 atrial flutter cycles. Thus, the correct diagnosis of this ECG tracing is atrial flutter with Wenckebach AV block (the AV conduction ratios alternate between 3:1 and 2:1).

The atrial flutter cycle (atrial rate: 200 beats/min) is slower than usual because of the quinidine effect. The therapeutic approach to atrial flutter has been described in Case 83. The atrial flutter waves are shown clearly in leads V_1 and II.

Left ventricular hypertrophy is suggested.

CASE 90

This ECG tracing was recorded from an 81-year-old man with cardiomyopathy. He has been taking digoxin 0.25 mg once and quinidine 0.2 g 4 times daily by mouth.

1. What is the cardiac rhythm diagnosis?

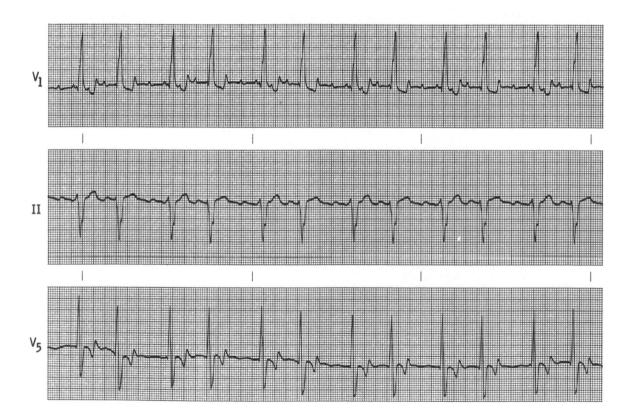

CASE 90: *Diagnosis*

The cardiac rhythm is atrial flutter (atrial rate: 230 beats/min) with Wenckebach AV block (ventricular rate: 75 beats/min). The ventricular cycle shows a regular irregularity, meaning that long and short R-R intervals alternate throughout the tracing. The short R-R interval is longer than 2 atrial flutter cycles, whereas the long R-R interval is shorter than 4 atrial flutter cycles. The long R-R interval is shorter than 2 short R-R intervals. Of course, F-R intervals (the interval from the last flutter wave to the next QRS complex) lengthen until the ventricular pause occurs. These findings are characteristic features of Wenckebach AV block (see Case 2). In this case, the AV conduction ratios vary between 2:1 and 4:1.

As repeatedly emphasized, slower than usual atrial flutter rate is most commonly due to the quinidine effect. The therapeutic approach to atrial flutter has been described in Case 83.

CASE 91

A 79-year-old woman with a permanent artificial pacemaker was examined at the pacemaker clinic at a follow-up visit. She complained of palpitations but was not taking any medication.
1. What is the cardiac rhythm diagnosis?
2. What is most likely the underlying disorder?
3. What is the proper therapeutic approach?

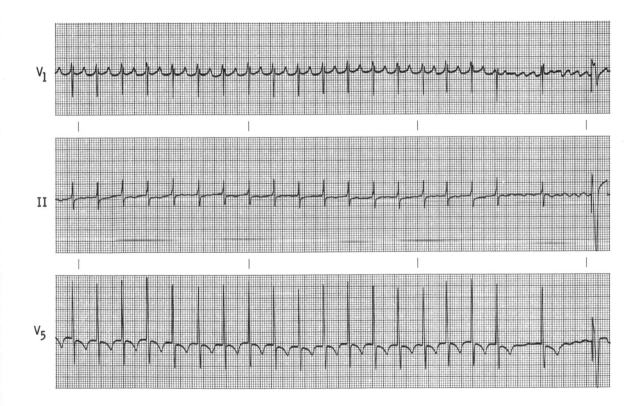

V₁

II

V₅

CASE 91: Diagnosis

The cardiac rhythm is atrial flutter (atrial rate: 272 beats/min) with 2:1 AV conduction, and intermittent atrial flutter–fibrillation with advanced AV block and 1 artificial pacemaker-induced ventricular beat. These ECG findings represent a form of bradytachyarrhythmias that is a manifestation of advanced SSS (see Case 52). A permanent artificial pacemaker was implanted for her advanced SSS.

As shown in this ECG tracing, atrial flutter with 2:1 AV conduction is not suppressed by the artificial pacing. Thus, digitalis or antiarrhythmic drug therapy (e.g., quinidine) is indicated because of her symptom (i.e., palpitations).

Note that there is left ventricular hypertrophy.

CASE 92

Cardiac consultation was requested on a 74-year-old woman because her cardiac rhythm was found to be very unstable and slow. She often experienced dizziness and near-syncope. She was not taking any medication.

1. What is the cardiac rhythm diagnosis?
2. What is most likely the underlying disorder?
3. What is the proper therapeutic approach?

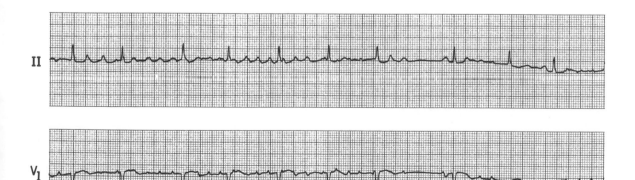

CASE 92: Diagnosis

The underlying rhythm is sinus (the 8th and 10th beats), but atrial flutter–fibrillation with advanced AV block occurs intermittently. This ECG finding is usually a manifestation of SSS (see Case 52). In this case, the sinus node is only partially functioning so that the ectopic atrial foci take over the cardiac activity whenever the sinus node fails to produce the cardiac impulses.

Holter monitor ECG is highly recommended in order to document various other manifestations of SSS (see Case 52) so that the indications vs nonindications of artificial pacing will be determined. When the Holter monitor ECG demonstrates markedly slow heart rhythm (usually slower than 40 beats/min) or a ventricular pause longer than 3 seconds, permanent artificial pacing is highly recommended. Electrophysiologic study (e.g., determination of the sinus node recovery time) should be performed if the Holter monitor ECG finding is equivocal.

CASE 93

A 63-year-old woman was seen at the cardiac clinic because of slow and irregular heart rhythm. She was not taking any medication and was relatively asymptomatic.
1. What is the cardiac rhythm diagnosis?
2. What is most likely the underlying disorder?
3. What is the proper therapeutic approach?

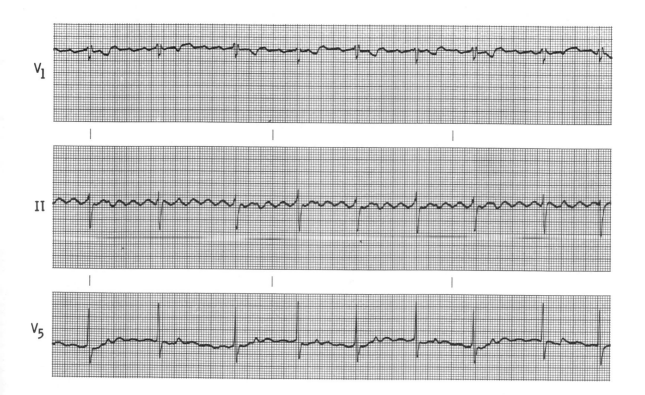

V₁

II

V₅

CASE 93: *Diagnosis*

The cardiac rhythm is atrial flutter (atrial rate: 260 beats/min) with advanced AV block, causing a slow and irregular ventricular cycle (ventricular rate: 50–55 beats/min). The ventricular cycle is irregular because the AV conduction ratios are not constant.

This ECG finding is most likely a manifestation of advanced SSS (see Case 52).

The therapeutic approach under this circumstance has been described in Case 92.

Other ECG abnormalities include incomplete RBBB and left anterior hemiblock.

Chapter 5
AV Junctional
Arrhythmias

CASE 94

These ECG rhythm strips were obtained from a 68-year-old man with a history of previous diaphragmatic MI and mild hypertension.
1. What is the cardiac rhythm diagnosis?
2. What is the ECG diagnosis?

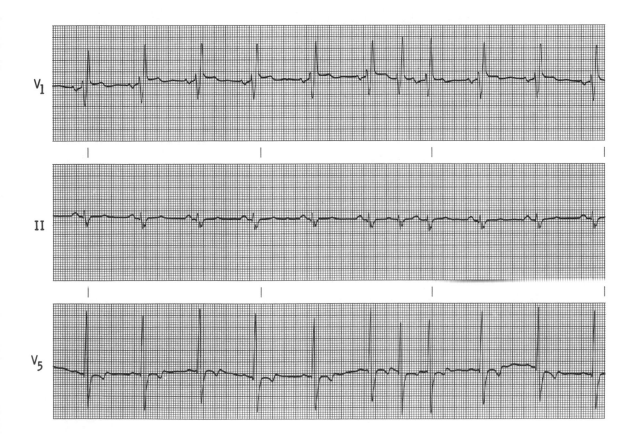

CASE 94: Diagnosis

The underlying cardiac rhythm is sinus (rate: 62 beats/min), but there is an interpolated AV junctional premature beat (the 7th beat). Note that the basic sinus P-P cycle is not disturbed and the ectopic beat has the same QRS configuration as the basic sinus beats. The P-R interval of the sinus beat immediately following the AV junctional premature beat is prolonged as a result of concealed AV conduction.

RBBB and left ventricular hypertrophy are obvious. In addition, left atrial hypertrophy is suggested. The evidence of old diaphragmatic MI is not clear in lead II (large Q waves in leads III and aVF—not shown here).

CASE 95

This ECG tracing was taken on a 55-year-old woman during a routine medical checkup. She was found to be asymptomatic, although her blood pressure was slightly elevated. She was not taking any medication.
1. What is the cardiac rhythm diagnosis?
2. Is there any other ECG abnormality?

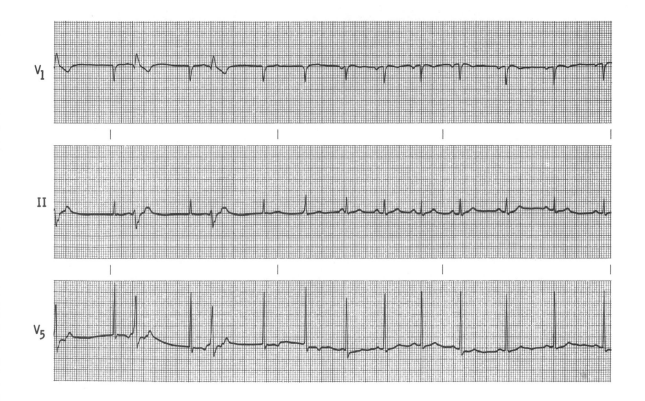

CASE 95: *Diagnosis*

The underlying cardiac rhythm is sinus arrhythmia with a rate of 70–85 beats/min (the latter half of tracing). Note that there are frequent VPCs causing ventricular bigeminy, and each VPC is followed by an AV junctional escape beat (the first half of tracing). In the mid-portion of the tracing, there are 3 consecutive AV junctional group beats (the 6th, 7th, and 8th beats) following a period of ventricular bigeminy.

Another interesting ECG finding in this tracing is the alteration of the T wave configuration in the AV junctional beats following VPCs. This T wave abnormality is termed "postectopic T wave change," which is nearly always found in patients with a diseased heart.

Holter monitor ECG is highly recommended in this patient in order to assess the nature and frequency of her ventricular ectopy.

Left ventricular hypertrophy is suggested.

CASE 96

An 83-year-old man was brought to the emergency room because of palpitations of acute onset. He was not taking any medication. He complained of weakness, but his vital signs were within normal limits except for a rapid pulse rate.
1. What is the cardiac rhythm diagnosis?
2. What is the proper therapeutic approach?

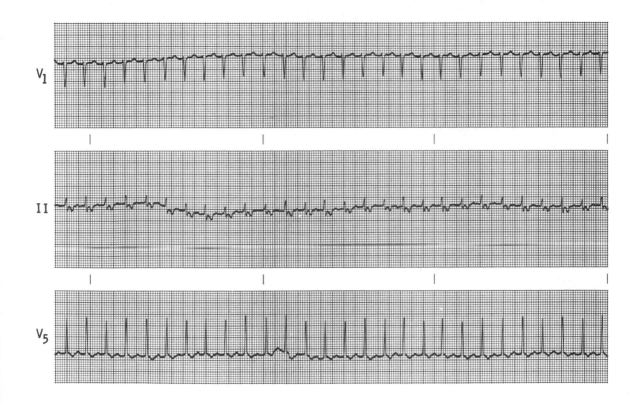

CASE 96: *Diagnosis*

The cardiac rhythm diagnosis is paroxysmal AV junctional tachycardia or reciprocating tachycardia with a rate of 175 beats/min. Note that each QRS complex is followed by a retrograde P wave, and the ventricular cycle is precisely regular with normal QRS complexes. The underlying mechanism responsible for the production of this tachycardia is considered to be a reentry phenomenon in the AV junction.

As far as the therapeutic approach is concerned, CSS is the first therapeutic step. As seen in paroxysmal atrial tachycardia (see Case 67), CSS is often effective in terminating paroxysmal AV junctional or reciprocating tachycardia. If CSS is ineffective, digitalization will be the next step (rapid method). Digitalis is also very effective in abolishing various supraventricular tachyarrhythmias. When digitalis is found to be ineffective, propranolol (Inderal) or verapamil may be tried. Electrophysiologic studies should be strongly considered when the above-mentioned common therapeutic approaches fail to terminate the tachycardia.

In addition, possible underlying causes (e.g., emotional stress, alcohol consumption, excessive intake of coffee or tea, hyperthyroidism, WPW syndrome, MVPS) should be investigated and eliminated (or controlled) if possible.

CASE 97

Digitalis toxicity was suspected on a 56-year-old hypertensive man with chronic CHF.
1. What is the cardiac rhythm diagnosis?
2. What other ECG abnormality is present?
3. Describe common causes of this arrhythmia.

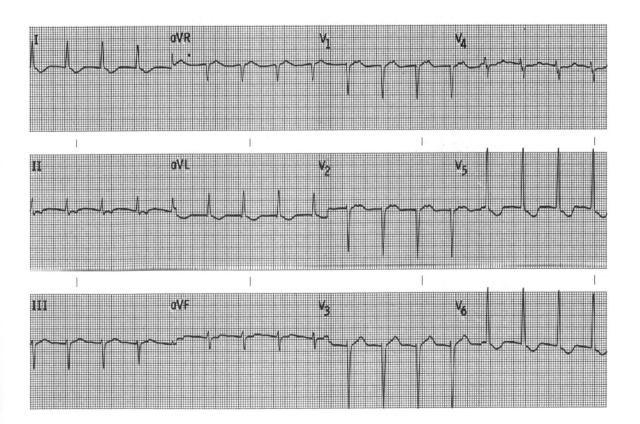

CASE 97: *Diagnosis*

The cardiac rhythm is nonparoxysmal AV junctional tachycardia with a rate of 100 beats/min. It should be noted that each QRS complex is followed by a retrograde P wave, and the ventricular cycle is regular with normal QRS complexes. The usual heart rate in nonparoxysmal AV junctional tachycardia ranges from 70 to 130 beats/min.

As far as the underlying causes of this arrhythmia are concerned, digitalis toxicity is the most common cause of nonparoxysmal AV junctional tachycardia. The next common cause is acute diaphragmatic (inferior) MI (see Case 105). Otherwise, nonparoxysmal AV junctional tachycardia may be observed during the immediate postoperative period following various cardiac operations (see Cases 98 and 99), in hypoxia due to various causes, and in myocarditis.

The diagnosis of left ventricular hypertrophy is obvious.

CASE 98

This ECG tracing was obtained from a 61-year-old woman soon after coronary artery bypass surgery. The surgery was said to be uneventful, and the patient's clinical condition was reported to be stable.
1. What is the cardiac rhythm diagnosis?
2. What is the proper therapeutic approach?

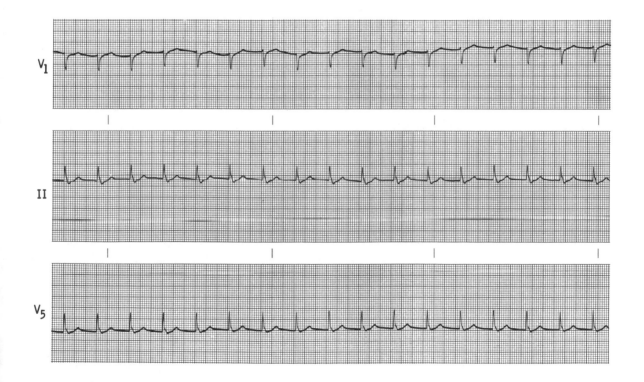

CASE 98: *Diagnosis*

The cardiac rhythm is nonparoxysmal AV junctional tachycardia with a rate of 98 beats/min. Note that all retrograde P waves are superimposed on the end portion (S waves) of the QRS complexes.

Postoperative nonparoxysmal AV junctional tachycardia is usually self-limited, and no treatment is necessary in most cases.

CASE 99

Aortic valve replacement was performed successfully on a 69-year-old woman, but her cardiac rhythm was changed postoperatively. Her clinical condition was said to be satisfactory and stable.

1. What is the cardiac rhythm diagnosis?
2. What is the proper therapeutic approach?

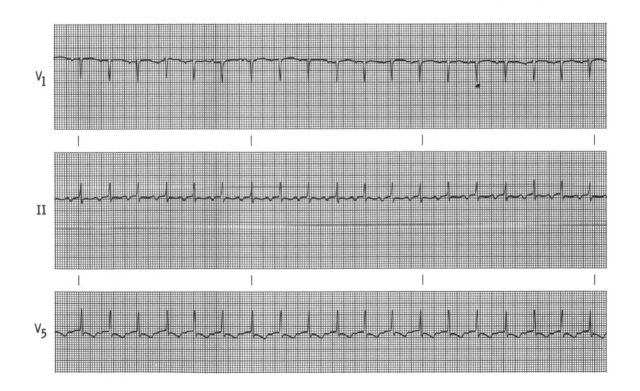

CASE 99: Diagnosis

The cardiac rhythm exhibits a regular tachycardia with a rate of 123 beats/min, and each QRS complex is preceded by a retrograde P wave with a relatively long P-R interval. The QRS configuration is normal.

Several possible mechanisms responsible for the production of this arrhythmia may be considered. The rhythm may be interpreted as nonparoxysmal AV junctional tachycardia with first degree AV block or reciprocating tachycardia. Otherwise, it may be diagnosed as coronary sinus tachycardia.

At any rate, most postoperative supraventricular tachycardias with a relatively slow rate do not cause a significant hemodynamic abnormality and are self-limited. Accordingly, no particular treatment is necessary in most cases.

CASE 100

This ECG tracing was taken on a 43-year-old, apparently healthy woman as a part of a routine medical checkup. There was no demonstrable heart disease, and she was not taking any medication.
1. What is the cardiac rhythm diagnosis?
2. What is the proper therapeutic approach?

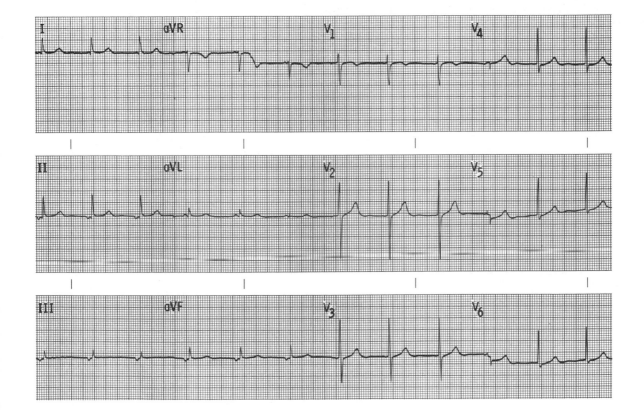

CASE 100: Diagnosis

The cardiac rhythm is nonparoxysmal AV junctional tachycardia with a rate of 70 beats/min. It should be noted that each QRS complex is preceded by a retrograde P wave and the QRS configuration is normal. The P-R interval is very short (0.08 second).

Although nonparoxysmal AV junctional tachycardia is commonly due to digitalis toxicity and acute diaphragmatic (inferior) MI, this arrhythmia may be observed in apparently healthy individuals on rare occasions. Under this circumstance, no treatment is necessary. Some investigators consider this arrhythmia in healthy people as an exaggerated form of sinus arrhythmia with wandering atrial pacemaker. At any rate, the finding is a benign arrhythmia.

CASE 101

An 82-year-old woman was seen at the cardiac clinic at a periodic medical checkup. Digitalis toxicity was suspected.

1. What is the cardiac rhythm diagnosis?

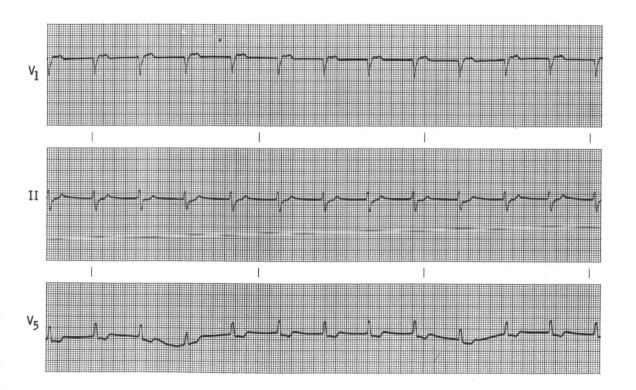

CASE 101: Diagnosis

The cardiac rhythm is nonparoxysmal AV junctional tachycardia with a rate of 74 beats/min. Note that the ventricular cycle is regular and some QRS complexes are followed by retrograde P waves (meaning intermittent atrial capture).

In AV junctional beats, a retrograde P wave may be preceded by or followed by a QRS complex, depending upon the sequence of the atrial and ventricular activation. When the atrial and ventricular activation occurs simultaneously, a retrograde P wave will be superimposed on the QRS complex, leading to absence of P waves. These atrial activation sequences in relation to the ventricular activation are insignificant clinically. Of course, the atrial and ventricular activation may be independent, leading to complete or incomplete AV dissociation (see Cases 104 and 105).

Incomplete LBBB is suggested.

CASE 102

A 60-year-old woman was referred to a cardiologist for evaluation of her cardiac arrhythmia. She was not taking any medication and was said to be apparently healthy and asymptomatic. She mentioned, however, that her heart rate seemed to be very slow from time to time in the past.

1. What is the cardiac rhythm diagnosis?
2. What is the proper therapeutic approach?

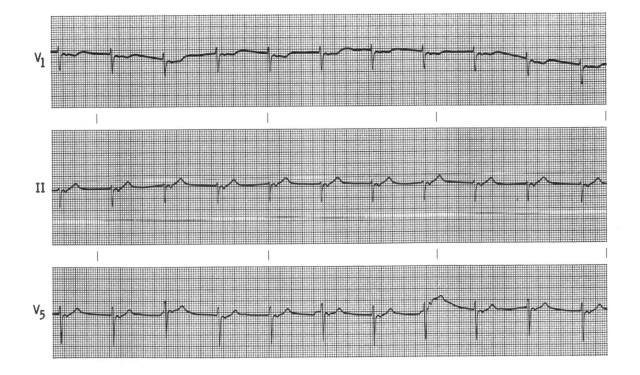

CASE 102: Diagnosis

The cardiac rhythm is nonparoxysmal AV junctional tachycardia with a rate of 67 beats/min. Note that each QRS complex is followed by a retrograde P wave, meaning that the AV junctional pacemaker activates the ventricles and the atria sequentially.

Although, by definition, the AV junctional escape rhythm has to be slower than 60 beats/min, it is not uncommon to observe that the AV junctional pacemaker may produce a different heart rate from time to time (sometimes faster or slower than 60 beats/min). Therefore, a heart rate slightly faster than 60 beats/min is often considered to be a slightly accelerated AV junctional escape rhythm.

When AV junctional escape rhythm persists without any specific reason (e.g., digitalis intoxication), especially in older adults, SSS should always be considered as a possible underlying disorder (see Case 52). Thus, the Holter monitor ECG is highly recommended in order to document other manifestations of SSS. When any ECG findings are suggestive of advanced SSS (e.g., very slow heart rate less than 40 beats/min, a long ventricular pause greater than 3 seconds), permanent artificial pacing should be strongly considered. Electrophysiologic study is recommended when the Holter monitor ECG findings are equivocal.

The diagnosis of left anterior hemiblock can be established without any difficulty.

CASE 103

A 69-year-old man has been taking digoxin 0.25 mg once and quinidine 0.3 g 4 times daily by mouth for several months for chronic CHF. Digitalis toxicity was suspected because a new cardiac arrhythmia was recorded and the patient's clinical condition was worse than before.
1. What is the cardiac rhythm diagnosis?
2. What other ECG abnormalities are present?

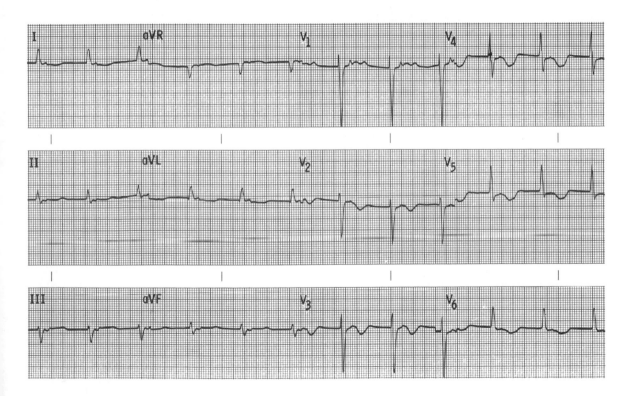

CASE 103: *Diagnosis*

The cardiac rhythm is nonparoxysmal AV junctional tachycardia with a rate of 68 beats/min. Note that each QRS complex is followed by a retrograde P wave.

Anterior myocardial ischemia is suggested on the basis of inverted T waves in practically all precordial leads. Another ECG abnormality is prolonged Q-T interval due to the quinidine effect. In addition, prominent U waves are compatible with hypokalemia.

It is well documented that hypokalemia and concomitant quinidine therapy predispose to digoxin toxicity.

Incomplete LBBB is diagnosed.

CASE 104

This ECG tracing was obtained from a 68-year-old woman with a long-standing CHF associated with chronic AF. She has been taking digoxin 0.25 mg and hydrochlorothiazide 50 mg daily by mouth. Digitalis intoxication was suspected because her cardiac rhythm had changed and her CHF seemed to be getting worse.

1. What is the cardiac rhythm diagnosis?
2. What other ECG abnormalities are present?
3. What is the proper therapeutic approach?

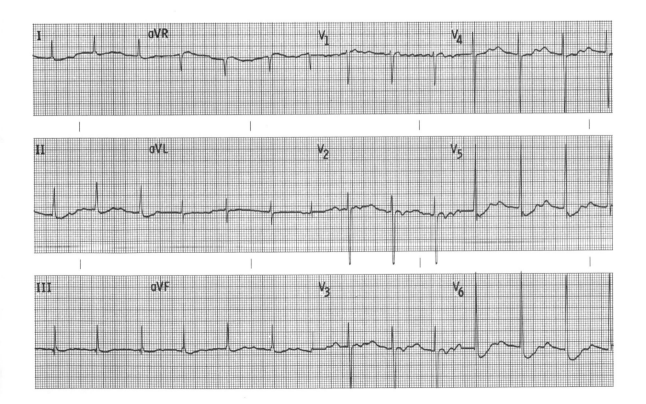

CASE 104: *Diagnosis*

The underlying cardiac rhythm is AF, but the R-R intervals are regular in most areas. The correct rhythm diagnosis, therefore, is AF with predominantly nonparoxysmal AV junctional tachycardia (rate: 80 beats/min), producing incomplete AV dissociation.

When nonparoxysmal AV junctional tachycardia develops in the presence of AF or atrial flutter, the direct cause is nearly always digitalis toxicity (see Case 97). It can be said that nonparoxysmal AV junctional tachycardia in the presence of AF is probably the most common digitalis-induced arrhythmia.

Other ECG abnormalities include left ventricular hypertrophy and prominent U waves indicative of hypokalemia.

Obviously, digitalis should be discontinued immediately when digitalis intoxication is diagnosed. In addition, potassium is often useful in the treatment of digitalis toxicity, especially when the serum potassium is found to be low. Remember that hypokalemia predisposes to digitalis toxicity.

CASE 105

A 46-year-old man was admitted to the CCU because of chest pain of 2 hours' duration. On admission to the CCU, his clinical status seemed to be stable, and his vital signs were found to be within normal limits. He was not taking any medication before this admission.

1. What is the cardiac rhythm diagnosis?
2. What is the ECG diagnosis?
3. What is the proper therapeutic approach?

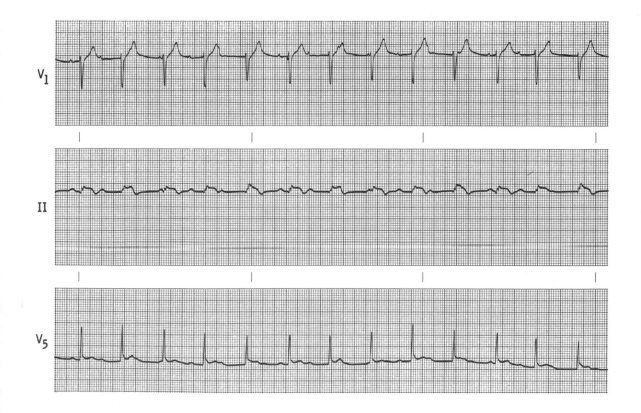

CASE 105: Diagnosis

The cardiac rhythm exhibits sinus tachycardia (atrial rate: 116 beats/min) with nonparoxysmal AV junctional tachycardia (ventricular rate: 83 beats/min), producing complete AV dissociation. Note that the atrial and the ventricular activities are independent throughout.

The diagnosis of acute diaphragmatic (inferior) MI can be readily made on the basis of pathologic Q waves in leads II, III, and aVF, associated with marked S-T segment elevation and T wave inversion (only lead II is shown here).

Various AV junctional arrhythmias and AV block of varying degrees often occur in acute diaphragmatic MI because the blood supply to the AV node is often impaired under this circumstance. However, these arrhythmias are usually transient and self-limited in most cases. Thus, no active treatment is necessary for nonparoxysmal AV junctional tachycardia associated with acute diaphragmatic MI.

Posterior myocardial ischemia (often associated with acute diaphragmatic MI) is suggested on the basis of a tall and upright T wave in lead V_1. In addition, the S-T segment is slightly elevated in lead V_5, indicative of lateral subepicardial injury (also a common coexisting abnormality).

CASE 106

A 70-year-old woman was presented to the weekly advanced ECG conference because the arrhythmia was thought to be somewhat unusual. Digitalis toxicity was considered to be the etiologic factor.
1. What is the cardiac rhythm diagnosis?
2. What is the mechanism of varying P wave configuration?

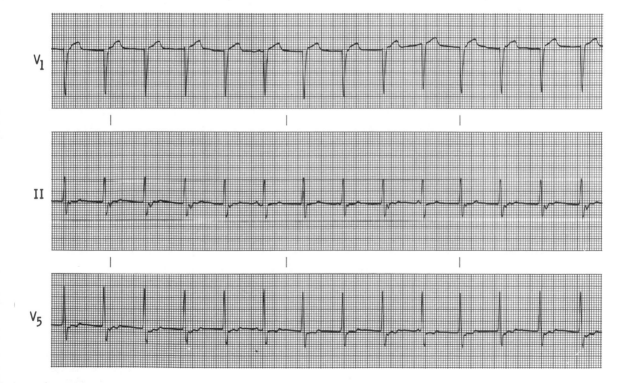

V_1

II

V_5

CASE 106: Diagnosis

The cardiac rhythm is nonparoxysmal AV junctional tachycardia (ventricular rate: 88 beats/min), but there are many different P waves. First, there are 3 upright P waves (most likely sinus in origin) unrelated to the QRS complexes (the P waves preceding the 6th, 8th, and 10th QRS complexes). In the remaining areas, each QRS complex is followed by a retrograde P wave of different configuration. This ECG finding indicates that the retrograde conduction from the AV junctional pacemaker to the atria varies from beat to beat. These findings, of course, are insignificant clinically.

Left ventricular hypertrophy is diagnosed.

CASE 107

This ECG tracing was taken on a 48-year-old man with rheumatic heart disease immediately following successful surgical replacement of the aortic valve for aortic insufficiency. His 12-lead ECG before the surgery was within normal limits other than left ventricular hypertrophy by voltage criteria. His postoperative course was reported to be uneventful and satisfactory.
1. What is the cardiac rhythm diagnosis?
2. What is the proper therapeutic approach?

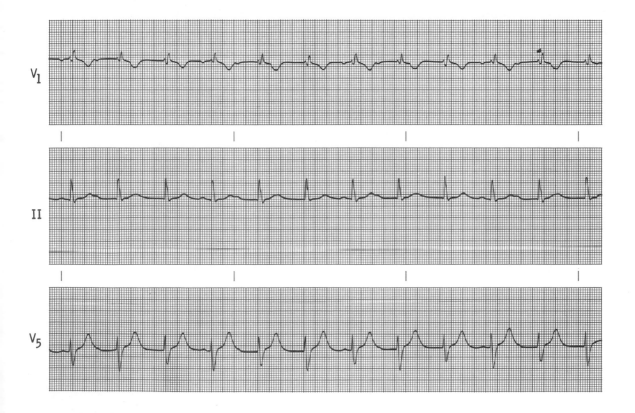

CASE 107: Diagnosis

The ventricular cycle is regular (rate: 74 beats/min) with RBBB pattern, but the QRS complex is relatively narrow. Thus, the cardiac rhythm diagnosis is sinus rhythm (atrial rate: 98 beats/min) with a fascicular tachycardia (rate: 74 beats/min), producing complete AV dissociation. It has been shown that the ectopic beat originating from one of the fascicles of the left bundle branch system shows incomplete RBBB pattern. In a broad sense, the fascicular tachycardia belongs to nonparoxysmal ventricular tachycardia. Remember that this patient did not have RBBB before the surgery. Alternatively, nonparoxysmal AV junctional tachycardia with a true incomplete RBBB is a possibility.

Fascicular tachycardia, nonparoxysmal ventricular tachycardia, and nonparoxysmal AV junctional tachycardia are not uncommon soon after various cardiac surgeries. These arrhythmias are usually self-limited and transient in most cases.

CASE 108

Cardiac consultation was requested on a 65-year-old woman with chronic AF because her cardiac rhythm appeared to be regular but the cardiac status seemed to be worse clinically than before. Digitalis intoxication was suspected immediately.
1. What is the cardiac rhythm diagnosis?
2. What other ECG abnormality is present?

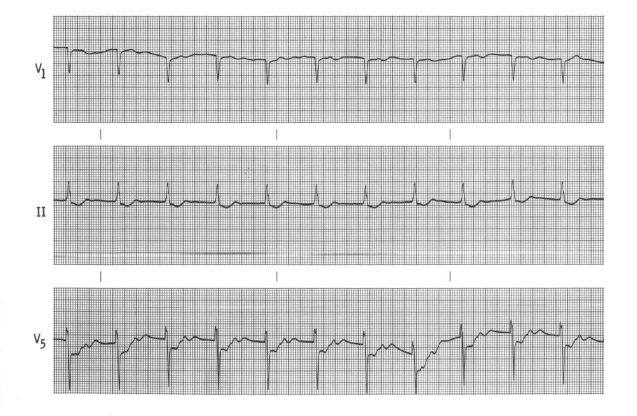

CASE 108: Diagnosis

The underlying cardiac rhythm is AF, but the ventricular cycle is regular throughout. Thus, the cardiac rhythm diagnosis is AF with nonparoxysmal AV junctional tachycardia (rate: 72 beats/min), producing complete AV dissociation. Note that the atrial and the ventricular activities are independent throughout the tracing.

It has been repeatedly emphasized that nonparoxysmal AV junctional tachycardia especially in the presence of AF is almost a pathognomonic feature of digitalis intoxication (see Cases 94 and 104).

Prominent U waves are readily recognized, particularly in lead V_5, and this ECG finding is indicative of hypokalemia. Hypokalemia, as previously described (see Case 104), frequently predisposes to digitalis toxicity.

CASE 109

A 57-year-old man with chronic CHF was referred to a cardiologist because a new cardiac arrhythmia was observed during oral maintenance digitalis therapy. He had had normal sinus rhythm previously.
1. What is the cardiac rhythm diagnosis?
2. What is the proper therapeutic approach?

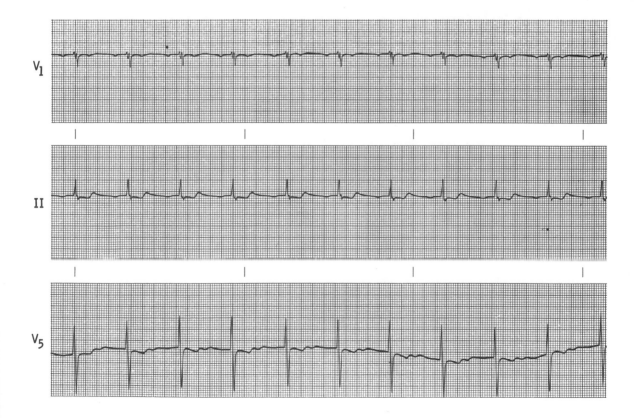

V_1

II

V_5

CASE 109: Diagnosis

Initially, the cardiac rhythm appears to be a regular sinus rhythm if the reader fails to recognize retrograde P waves. By close observation, however, experienced readers should be able to appreciate regularly occurring retrograde P waves. There are 2 retrograde P waves between each R-R interval. The correct diagnosis is nonparoxysmal AV junctional tachycardia (atrial rate: 130 beats/min) with 2:1 AV block. Note that every other retrograde P wave is not conducted to the ventricles because of forward (antegrade) block from the AV junctional pacemaker to the ventricles on every other cardiac impulse. In other words, this ECG finding is 2:1 unidirectional exit block (forward or antegrade conduction). Inexperienced readers may easily fail to recognize every other retrograde P wave that is superimposed on the early portion of the T wave.

Digitalis toxicity was diagnosed, and the drug was discontinued immediately. Prominent U waves are suggestive of hypokalemia (see Cases 104 and 108).

CASE 110

Because of the interesting features of her cardiac arrhythmia, a 63-year-old woman was presented to the weekly cardiology conference. Digitalis toxicity was considered to be an etiologic factor of her cardiac arrhythmia.
1. What is the cardiac rhythm diagnosis?
2. What other ECG abnormality is present?

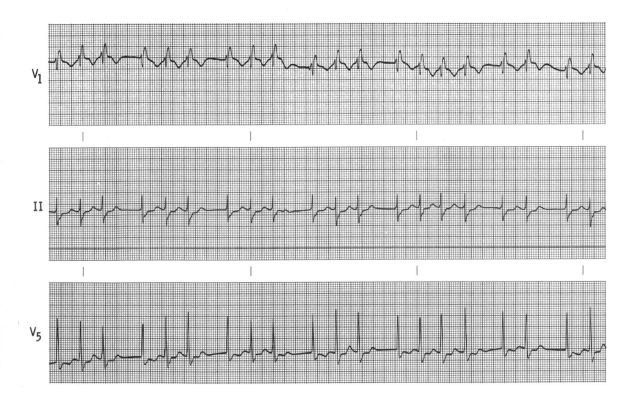

V₁

II

V₅

CASE 110: Diagnosis

There are no discernible P waves, but the ventricular cycles are not grossly irregular. Therefore, the cardiac rhythm is not a simple AF. One can appreciate that 2–4 ventricular group beats are followed by long ventricular pauses. The long ventricular pause is less than 2 short R-R intervals. In addition, the long R-R intervals are almost equal to each other in duration. By careful observation, experienced readers may be able to appreciate the progressive shortening of the R-R intervals during the ventricular group beating in most areas. When these electrophysiologic events are analyzed together, the correct rhythm diagnosis of this tracing is AF and nonparoxysmal AV junctional tachycardia (rate: 147 beats/min) with Wenckebach exit block of varying degree, producing complete AV dissociation.

Another ECG abnormality is, obviously, RBBB.

CASE 111

These ECG rhythm strips were obtained from a 36-year-old healthy woman at a routine test.
1. What is the cardiac rhythm diagnosis?
2. What is the proper therapeutic approach?

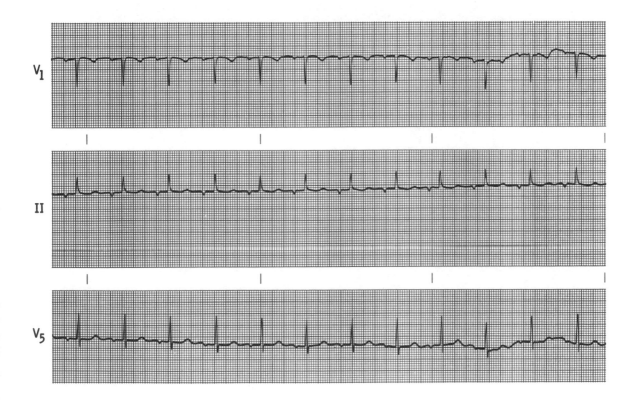

CASE 111: Diagnosis

The cardiac rhythm diagnosis is coronary sinus rhythm with a rate of 78 beats/min. The P waves are found to be inverted in leads II, III, aVF, and V_{5-6} (only leads II and V_5 are shown here).

The diagnosis of coronary sinus rhythm is established when the P waves are inverted in all inferior leads (meaning the P axis ranging from −60 to −90 degrees) and the P-R interval is longer than 0.12 second (between 0.12 and 0.20 second). Leads V_{4-6} may show upright, inverted, or biphasic (or flat) P waves in coronary sinus rhythm. The P waves in leads V_{1-2} usually exhibit biphasic configuration under this circumstance.

Clinically, coronary sinus rhythm is considered to be a benign arrhythmia, and, accordingly, no treatment is needed.

CASE 112

A 70-year-old man was referred to the cardiac clinic because his cardiac rhythm was found to be very slow and there were several episodes of near-syncope. He was not taking any medication.
1. What is the cardiac rhythm diagnosis?
2. What is most likely the underlying cardiac disorder?
3. What is the proper therapeutic approach?

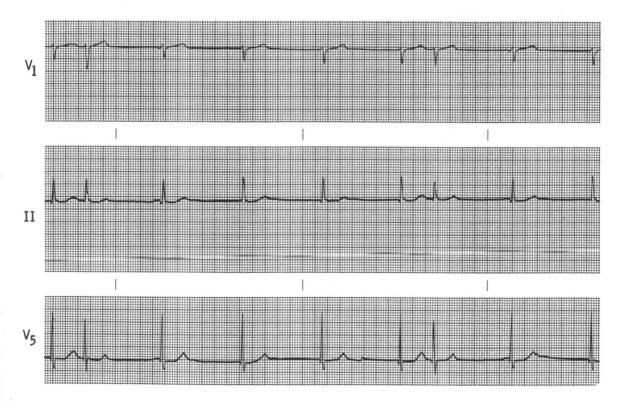

V₁

II

V₅

CASE 112: Diagnosis

The cardiac rhythm diagnosis is marked sinus bradycardia (atrial rate: 43 beats/min) with intermittent AV junctional escape rhythm (rate: 48 beats/min), producing incomplete AV dissociation. Note that the sinus P waves are independent of the QRS complexes except that there are 2 conducted sinus beats (ventricular captured beats—the 2nd and 7th beats). Both sinus beats show a slightly deformed configuration because of aberrant ventricular conduction.

As far as the underlying disorder is concerned, SSS is most likely responsible, and Holter monitor ECG is highly recommended to document other signs of advanced SSS (see Case 52). Permanent artificial pacing is indicated for all patients with symptomatic or advanced SSS.

CASE 113

A 56-year-old woman was examined at a cardiologist's office for the evaluation of her cardiac arrhythmia. She was asymptomatic and not taking any medication.
1. What is the cardiac rhythm diagnosis?
2. What is the proper therapeutic approach?

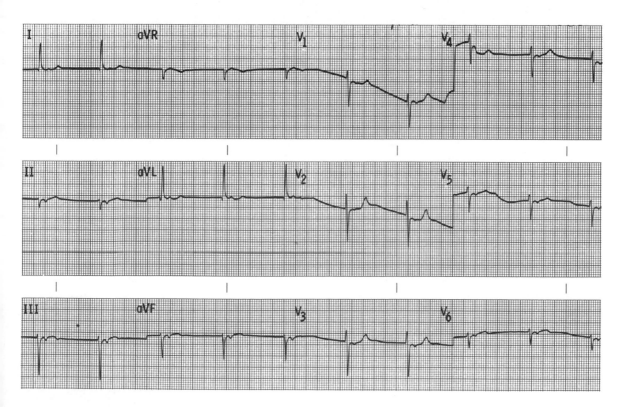

CASE 113: Diagnosis

The cardiac cycle is precisely regular with a rate of 55 beats/min, and each QRS complex is followed by a retrograde P wave. All QRS complexes are normal (narrow). Thus, the cardiac rhythm diagnosis is AV junctional escape rhythm (rate: 55 beats/min). In this case, the ventricles and the atria are activated sequentially by the AV junctional pacemaker. As described previously, each QRS complex may be preceded by or followed by a retrograde P wave in AV junctional tachycardia or escape rhythm.

Since the patient is found to be entirely asymptomatic, no active treatment is necessary. However, Holter monitor ECG is highly recommended for possible documentation of various ECG manifestations of advanced SSS (see Case 52). If any ECG finding indicative of advanced SSS (e.g., markedly slow escape rhythm less than 40 beats/min or sinus arrest or ventricular standstill longer than 3 seconds) is recorded in the Holter monitor ECG, permanent artificial pacing is strongly considered (see Case 52).

Left anterior hemiblock is diagnosed (QRS axis: −45 degrees).

CASE 114

A 74-year-old woman was admitted to the CCU because of a recent heart attack. She was apparently healthy until this admission and not taking any medication.
1. What is the cardiac rhythm diagnosis?
2. What is the proper therapeutic approach?

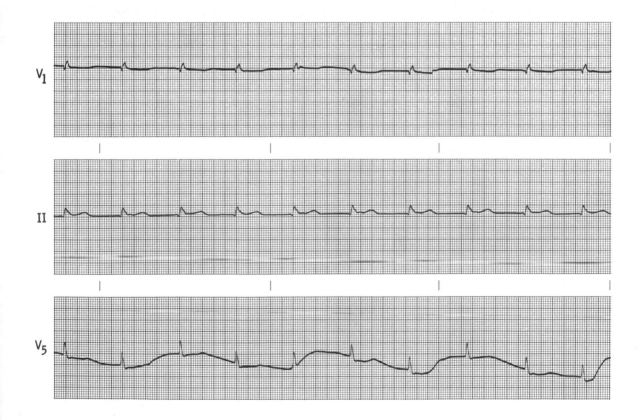

CASE 114: *Diagnosis*

The cardiac rhythm diagnosis is AV junctional escape rhythm with a rate of 58 beats/min. The cardiac cycle is precisely regular, but P waves are not discernible. It is a good possibility that the atrial mechanism may be AF.

No active treatment will be necessary under this circumstance as long as the arrhythmia causes no significant hemodynamic abnormality or symptom. Generally, AV junctional escape rhythm with reasonably fast ventricular rate (rate: 45–60 beats/min) does not produce any hemodynamic alteration.

Various AV junctional arrhythmias and AV block are common in recent diaphragmatic MI (see Cases 2, 5, and 13) secondary to impairment of the blood supply to the AV node. However, these arrhythmias are transient and self-limited in most cases. Thus, no active treatment is necessary.

Incomplete RBBB is diagnosed in addition to recent diaphragmatic MI.

CASE 115

Cardiac consultation was requested on a 69-year-old man because his pulse rate was found to be very slow. He complained of frequent episodes of dizziness and near-syncope. He was not taking any medication.

1. What is the cardiac rhythm diagnosis?
2. What is the proper therapeutic approach?

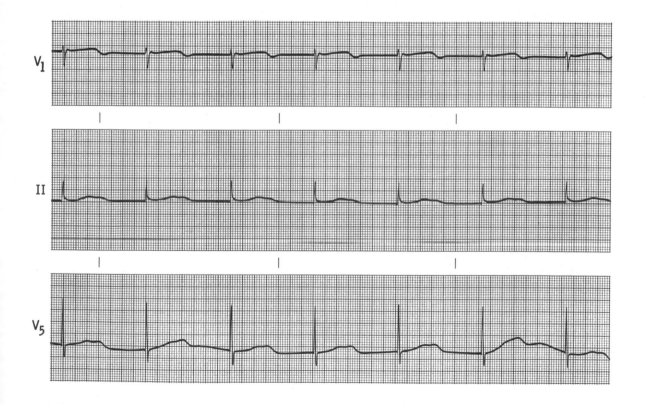

CASE 115: Diagnosis

No P waves are discernible, and the ventricular cycle is precisely regular. The QRS complexes are normal (narrow). Thus, the cardiac rhythm diagnosis is AV junctional escape rhythm with a rate of 43 beats/min.

When dealing with persisting AV junctional escape rhythm with or without intermittent sinus rhythm, a possibility of advanced SSS must always be considered as underlying disorder (see Case 52). In addition, Holter monitor ECG is highly recommended in order to document other ECG manifestations of advanced SSS. Permanent artificial pacing is indicated for symptomatic or advanced SSS.

Note the markedly prolonged Q-T interval, which is not uncommon among elderly people.

CASE 116

A 74-year-old man was evaluated at the cardiac clinic because he complained of weakness and dizziness associated with slow heart rate. He was not taking any drug.
1. What is the cardiac rhythm diagnosis?
2. What is the proper therapeutic approach?

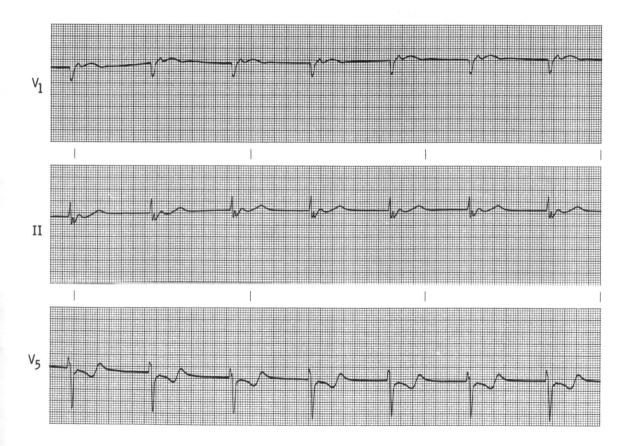

CASE 116: Diagnosis

The cardiac rhythm exhibits AV junctional escape rhythm with a rate of 44 beats/min. Note that each QRS complex is followed by a retrograde P wave.

SSS is most likely responsible for the production of this arrhythmia (see Cases 52 and 115). The therapeutic approach to SSS was described in Case 115.

Another ECG abnormality in this tracing is prolonged Q-T interval, which is common in elderly individuals. The QRS complex appears to be very broad because a retrograde P wave is superimposed on the end portion of each QRS complex.

Chapter 6
Ventricular Arrhythmias

CASE 117

A 67-year-old man with a history of a heart attack 6 months previously visited his family physician's office for a follow-up examination. He was not taking any medication except for aspirin.
1. What is the cardiac rhythm diagnosis?
2. What is the proper therapeutic approach?

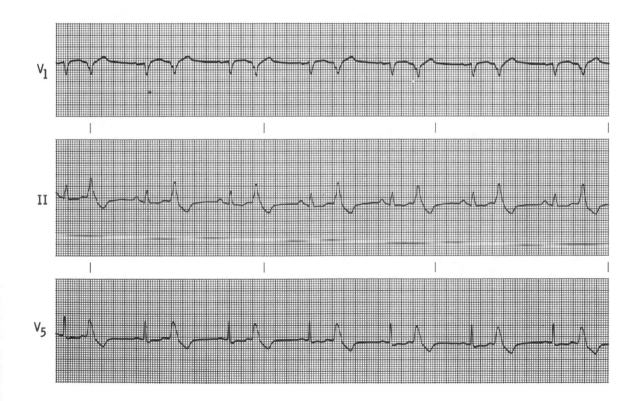

CASE 117: Diagnosis

The underlying cardiac rhythm is sinus with a rate of 84 beats/min. Note that there are frequent VPCs producing ventricular bigeminy. All VPCs have the identical configuration, meaning unifocal in origin. As a rule, the coupling interval (the interval from the ectopic beat to the preceding sinus beat) is constant when dealing with the ordinary VPC. In contrast, parasystole shows varying coupling intervals.

In the following situations, VPCs are considered to be clinically significant, and active treatment may be necessary in most cases.

Clinically Significant VPCs

1. Thirty or more VPCs per hour
2. Multifocal VPCs (see Case 124)
3. Grouped (2–5 beats in a row) VPCs (see Cases 125 and 126)
4. VPC with the R-on-T phenomenon (VPC superimposed on the top of the T wave of the preceding beat—see Case 120)
5. VPCs induced by exercise
6. VPCs immediately following termination of ventricular tachycardia or fibrillation

In general, Holter monitor ECG is highly recommended under this circumstance in order to assess the nature and the frequency of VPCs. Active treatment is most likely indicated when the VPCs are symptomatic (e.g., palpitations) or when the VPCs are found in patients with active or acute heart disease (e.g., acute MI). In other words, VPCs found in apparently healthy individuals are usually benign and require no active treatment.

CASE 118

This ECG tracing was obtained from a 70-year-old man. There was no particular complaint, and he was not taking any drug.
1. What is the cardiac rhythm diagnosis?
2. What is the proper therapeutic approach?
3. What other ECG abnormalities are present?

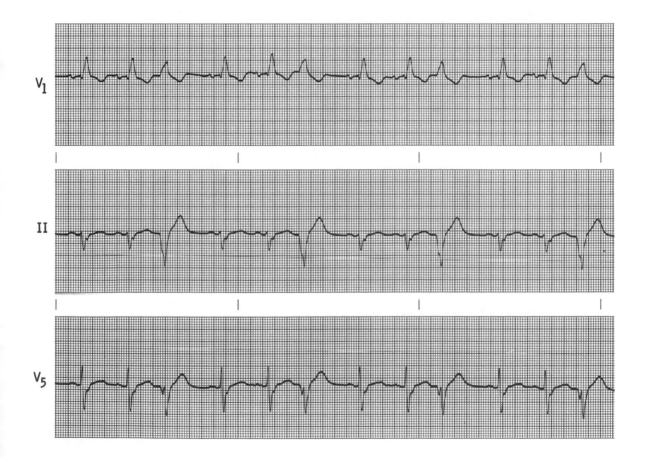

CASE 118: Diagnosis

The underlying cardiac rhythm is sinus with a rate of 80 beats/min. There are frequent VPCs, producing ventricular trigeminy, meaning that VPCs occur on every 3rd beat. These are unifocal in origin.

The proper therapeutic approach to VPCs has been described in Case 117.

Other ECG abnormalities include RBBB and left anterior hemiblock, causing BFB. In addition, left atrial hypertrophy is suggested.

CASE 119

A 48-year-old woman was evaluated at the cardiac clinic because of frequent extrasystoles. She was not taking any medication.
1. What is the cardiac rhythm diagnosis?
2. What is the proper diagnostic workup when dealing with extrasystoles?

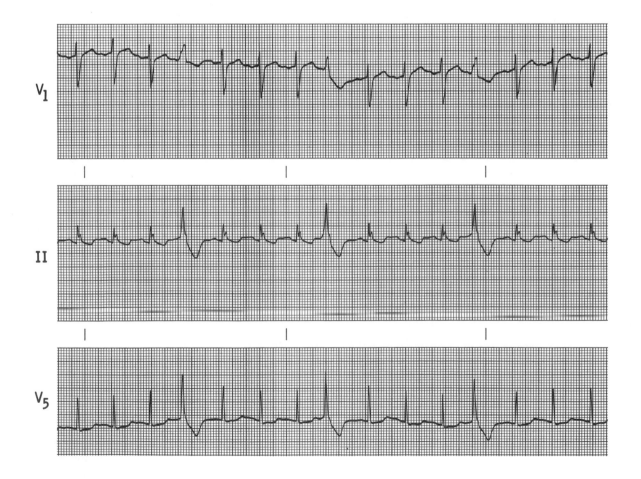

V₁

II

V₅

CASE 119: Diagnosis

The underlying cardiac rhythm is sinus tachycardia with a rate of 110 beats/min. There are frequent VPCs, producing ventricular quadrigeminy, meaning that VPCs occur on every 4th beat.

When dealing with any cardiac arrhythmia (e.g., VPCs, paroxysmal AF), one should investigate whether a given individual has any unusual personal habit (e.g., heavy smoking, excessive consumption of coffee, tea, cola drinks, or alcohol, emotional stress). If any of these contributing factors are found, they should be controlled or eliminated. When no contributing factor is found, however, other common disorders that frequently produce various cardiac arrhythmias should be investigated. For example, hyperthyroidism and MVPS should be tested for when dealing with any cardiac arrhythmia due to unknown cause.

Clinically significant VPCs were described in Case 117.

CASE 120

An 82-year-old woman with known CAD was examined at a cardiologist's office because of her cardiac arrhythmia. She was not taking any medication.

1. What is the cardiac rhythm diagnosis?
2. What is the proper therapeutic approach?

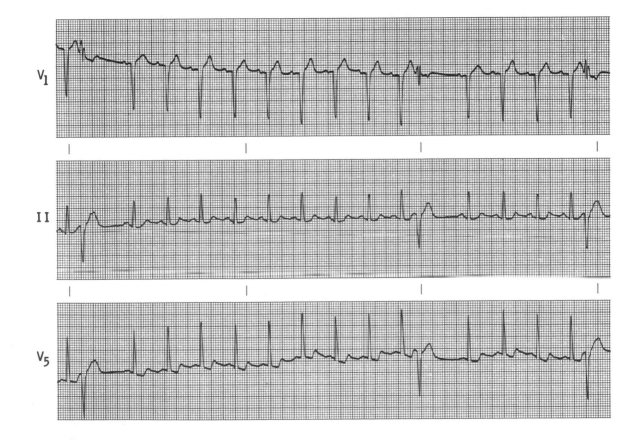

CASE 120: Diagnosis

The underlying cardiac rhythm is sinus tachycardia (rate: 105 beats/min), but there are frequent VPCs. It should be noted that the coupling interval is so short that the VPC is superimposed on the top of the T wave (the R-on-T phenomenon). As described in Case 117, the VPC with the R-on-T phenomenon is clinically significant and potentially serious, since ventricular fibrillation is easily provoked under this circumstance because the ventricular ectopic impulse is fired during the vulnerable period of the ventricles (the R-on-T phenomenon). Thus, the VPC with R-on-T phenomenon should be aggressively suppressed using the most effective antiarrhythmic agent (e.g., quinidine, procainamide) for a given patient.

The diagnosis of left ventricular hypertrophy is made without any difficulty.

CASE 121

This ECG tracing was recorded on a 62-year-old woman who complained of "skipped heart beats." She was not taking any medication.
1. What is the cardiac rhythm diagnosis?
2. What is most likely the origin of these ectopic beats?

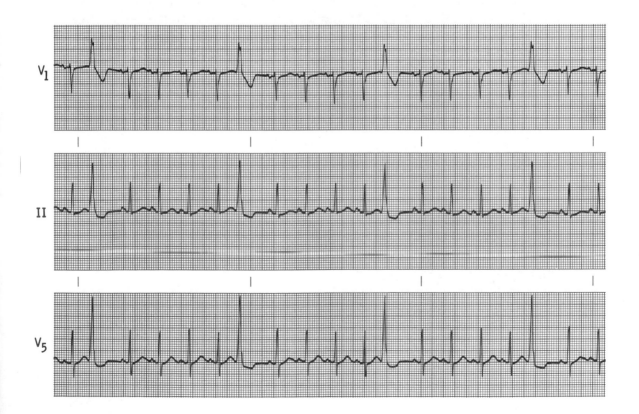

CASE 121: Diagnosis

The underlying cardiac rhythm is sinus tachycardia with a rate of 118 beats/min. Note that there are frequent VPCs that occur on every 5th beat.

Although the precise origin of the VPCs cannot be determined on a 12-lead ECG, the origin of the ectopic impulse formation may be assessed with reasonable certainty. For example, the VPCs originating from the right ventricle usually reveal negative QRS complexes in the right precordial leads and positive QRS complexes in the left precordial leads (see Case 117). Conversely, the left VPCs demonstrate upright QRS complexes in the right precordial leads and negative QRS complexes in the left precordial leads (see Cases 118 and 120). On the other hand, the QRS complexes are upright in both right and left precordial leads when VPCs arise from the ventricular septum, as seen in this patient.

Generally, VPCs found in healthy young individuals are commonly of right ventricular origin. VPCs arising from the left ventricle and the ventricular septum are more commonly encountered in elderly people and cardiac patients.

CASE 122

A 75-year-old man was examined at the cardiac clinic as a periodic medical checkup. He was not taking any drug.
1. What is the cardiac rhythm diagnosis?
2. What other ECG abnormality is present?

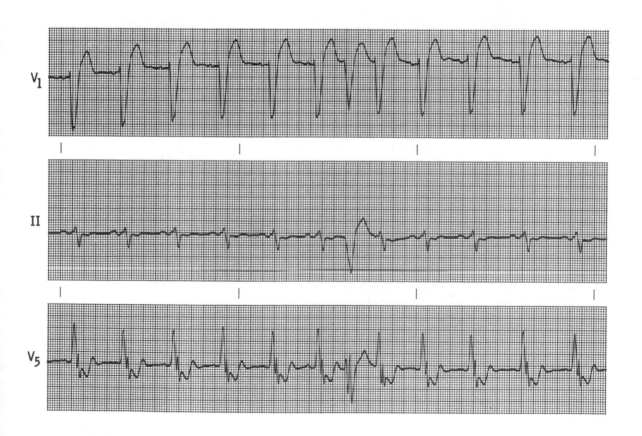

CASE 122: Diagnosis

The underlying cardiac rhythm is sinus with a rate of 73 beats/min. There are 2 ectopic beats, an APC (the 6th beat), followed by an interpolated VPC (the 7th beat).

The term "interpolated" VPC is used when a VPC is sandwiched between 2 consecutively appearing sinus beats without any pause. The R-R interval that contains an interpolated VPC is longer than the basic R-R interval simply because the P-R interval of the sinus beat immediately following the VPC is prolonged as a result of concealed ventriculoatrial conduction. In this ECG tracing, an APC precedes the interpolated VPC.

The diagnosis of LBBB is obvious. In addition, left atrial hypertrophy is also considered.

CASE 123

This ECG tracing was obtained from a 25-year-old woman with no demonstrable heart disease.
1. What is the cardiac rhythm diagnosis?
2. What is the clinical significance of this arrhythmia?

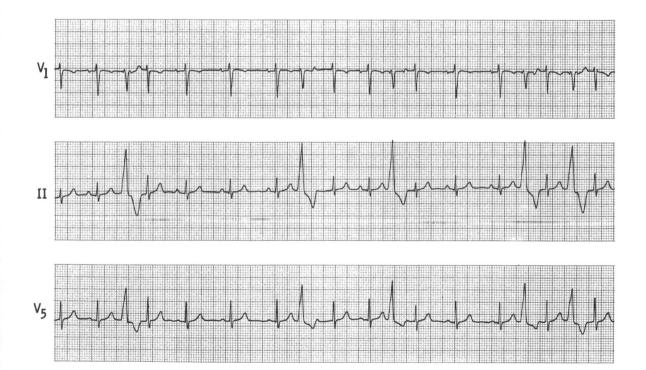

CASE 123: Diagnosis

The underlying cardiac rhythm is sinus arrhythmia (rate: 78–90 beats/min), but there are frequent VPCs. It should be noted that all VPCs are interpolated. These VPCs most likely originate from the right ventricle because the QRS complex of the ectopic beat is negative in lead V_1 and upright in lead V_5.

Generally, interpolated VPCs are benign arrhythmia, and the VPCs arising from the right ventricle are considered to be also benign arrhythmia.

CASE 124

A 59-year-old man with a history of diaphragmatic (inferior) MI 1 year previously was seen at a cardiologist's office as a follow-up medical checkup. He was not taking any medication.
1. What is the cardiac rhythm diagnosis?
2. What is the proper therapeutic approach?
3. What other ECG abnormality is present?

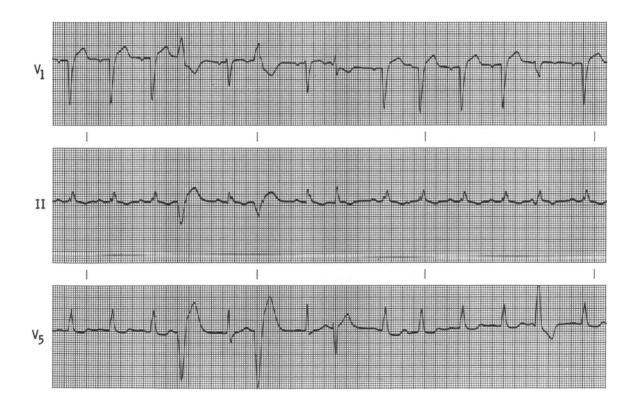

CASE 124: Diagnosis

The underlying cardiac rhythm is sinus (rate: 85 beats/min), but there are frequent multifocal VPCs. As described in Case 117, multifocal VPCs are considered to be clinically significant, and active antiarrhythmic drug therapy is indicated. Holter monitor ECG is highly recommended to assess the nature and the frequency of the ventricular ectopy. In addition, there is an APC (the 10th beat).

Another ECG abnormality is intermittent LBBB. In addition, left atrial hypertrophy is suggested.

CASE 125

A 68-year-old woman with known CAD was evaluated because of her cardiac arrhythmia. She had suffered from diaphragmatic MI 2 months previously, but her recovery was said to be uneventful. She was not taking any medication.

1. What is the cardiac rhythm diagnosis?
2. What is the proper therapeutic approach?

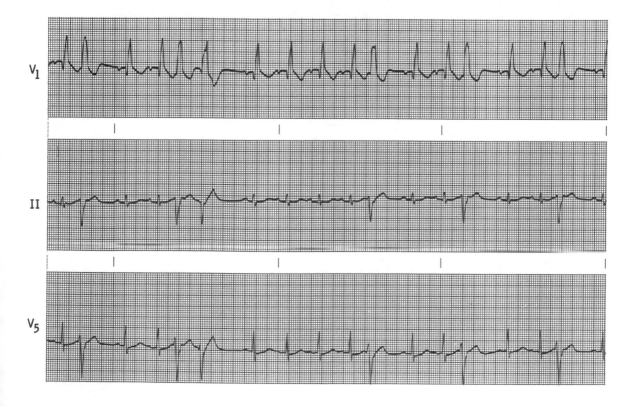

CASE 125: Diagnosis

The underlying cardiac rhythm is sinus tachycardia with a rate of 102 beats/min. Note that there are frequent VPCs with ventricular group beats (2 beats in a row) and the R-on-T phenomenon.

As described in Case 117, her ventricular ectopy is clinically significant and potentially serious, especially in view of her relatively recent MI. Thus, her VPCs should be aggressively treated with all available antiarrhythmic agents (e.g., quinidine, procainamide).

It is highly advisable to obtain a Holter monitor ECG in order to assess the exact nature and frequency of her ventricular ectopy. In addition, periodic follow-up Holter monitor ECGs should be taken to determine the efficacy of the antiarrhythmic drug therapy.

The diagnosis of RBBB is obvious, but diaphragmatic MI cannot be diagnosed with certainty when only these 3 ECG leads are available.

CASE 126

A 60-year-old man was admitted to the CCU because of an acute coronary event. He was not taking any medication before admission. Tracing A was taken on admission, and tracing B was obtained several hours later.
1. What is the cardiac rhythm diagnosis?
2. What is the proper therapeutic approach?
3. What is the ECG diagnosis?

A

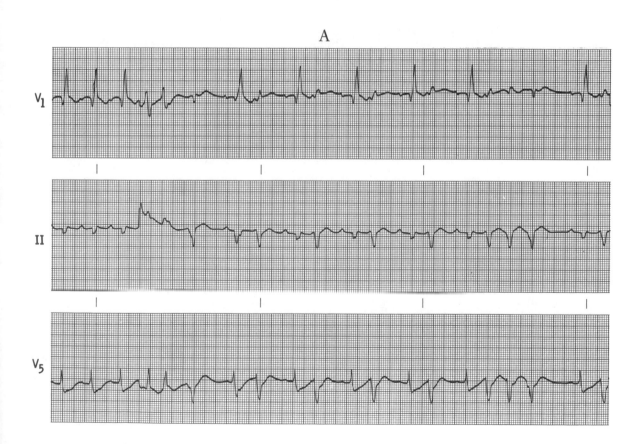

CASE 126: Diagnosis

Tracing A

The underlying cardiac rhythm is sinus tachycardia (rate: 113 beats/min) with first degree AV block. There are frequent VPCs with group beats (3 beats in a row), indicating potentially serious ventricular arrhythmia (see Case 117). The drug of choice for frequent VPCs, especially in the presence of acute MI, is intravenous injection of lidocaine (Xylocaine) followed by intravenous infusion.

Tracing B

Tracing B taken several hours later shows complete suppression of the ventricular ectopy by lidocaine administration.

There are several ECG abnormalities, including acute diaphragmatic (inferior) MI, anteroseptal MI, and RBBB. The underlying cardiac rhythm is sinus tachycardia (rate: 110 beats/min) with first degree AV block. Prophylactic artificial cardiac pacing is not indicated for RBBB associated with acute MI.

B

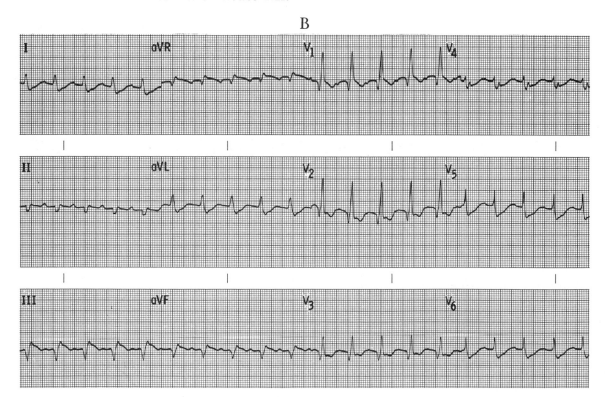

CASE 127

This ECG tracing was recorded on a 79-year-old woman with chronic CHF. Digitalis toxicity was suspected, and she was admitted to the intermediate cardiac care unit.
1. What is the cardiac rhythm diagnosis?
2. What is the proper therapeutic approach?

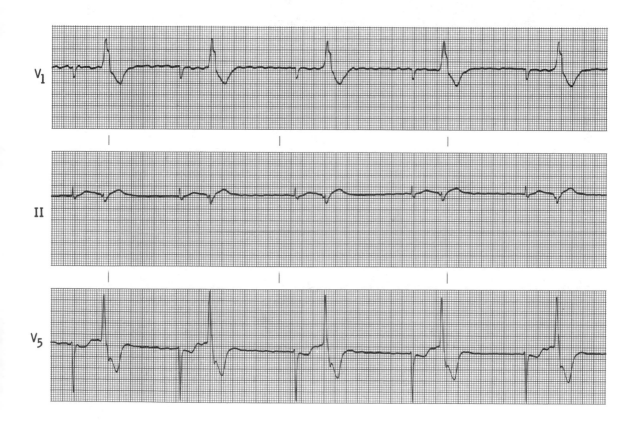

CASE 127: Diagnosis

The underlying cardiac rhythm is AF, but the ventricular rate is very slow. Thus, the rhythm diagnosis is AF with advanced (high degree) AV block, producing intermittent AV junctional escape beats (ventricular rate: 45–55/min) and frequent VPCs, causing ventricular bigeminy. When dealing with this type of cardiac arrhythmia during digitalis therapy, the diagnosis of digitalis toxicity is almost certain. The patient's serum digoxin level was found to be significantly elevated (serum digoxin level: 3.8 ng/ml).

Obviously, the first therapeutic approach to digitalis toxicity is immediate discontinuation of digitalis administration. When any digitalis-induced bradyarrhythmia causes significant hemodynamic abnormality (e.g., hypotension) or symptom (e.g., near-syncope), a temporary artificial cardiac pacing should be considered. In most cases, however, discontinuation of digitalis alone is sufficient. When VPCs persist even after withdrawal of digitalis, administration of potassium or phenytoin (Dilantin) may be indicated.

CASE 128

A 65-year-old man was brought to the emergency room because of rapid heart action with acute onset. He was not taking any medication.
1. What is the cardiac rhythm diagnosis?
2. What is the proper therapeutic approach?

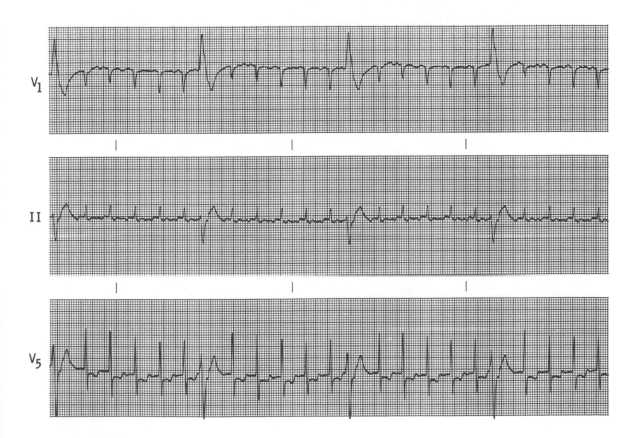

CASE 128: Diagnosis

The underlying cardiac rhythm is atrial flutter with 2:1 AV response (ventricular rate: 143 beats/min). There are frequent VPCs, which occur on every 6th beat, leading to a regular irregularity of the ventricular cycle.

The drug of choice for atrial flutter with 2:1 AV response is rapid digitalization (see Case 81). When the clinical situation is extremely urgent, however, immediate application of DC shock will be the treatment of choice. When VPCs persist, various antiarrhythmic drugs may be tried (e.g., quinidine, procainamide, lidocaine).

CASE 129

A 67-year-old woman was admitted to the CCU because of acute coronary event associated with a rapid heart action and hypotension. She was not taking any medication before admission.

1. What is the cardiac rhythm diagnosis?
2. What is the proper therapeutic approach?

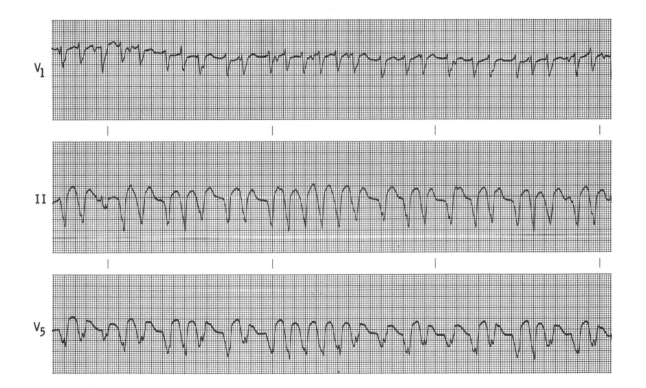

V₁

II

V₅

CASE 129: Diagnosis

The cardiac rhythm appears to be grossly irregular, and the QRS complexes are extremely bizarre. By close observation, experienced readers should be able to recognize regularly occurring P waves with a rate of 92 beats/min. Thus, sinus rhythm is present in the atria. The ventricular cycle is regular in some areas, with a rate of 200 beats/min. In some other areas, the longer R-R intervals are equal to each other. Thus, the complete cardiac rhythm diagnosis is sinus rhythm with multifocal ventricular tachycardia, producing AV dissociation.

The treatment of choice is immediate application of DC shock. When ventricular tachycardia is terminated, continuous intravenous lidocaine infusion is indicated for at least 2–3 days. Later, oral antiarrhythmic drug therapy will replace intravenous lidocaine infusion.

Holter monitor ECG is highly recommended before discharge to make certain that the patient's ventricular arrhythmia is properly controlled.

CASE 130

Digitalis toxicity was suspected in a 55-year-old woman.
1. What is the cardiac rhythm diagnosis?

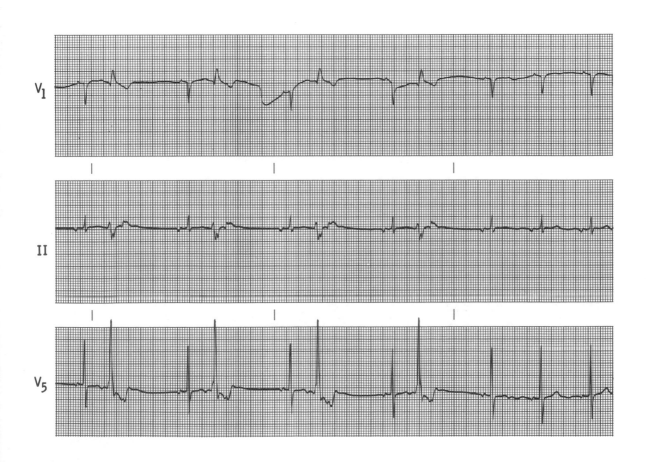

CASE 130: Diagnosis

The underlying cardiac rhythm is nonparoxysmal AV junctional tachycardia (rate: 73 beats/min), but there are frequent VPCs, producing ventricular bigeminy. These ECG findings are the characteristic feature of digitalis toxicity.

Various aspects of digitalis-induced nonparoxysmal AV junctional tachycardia have been discussed in Cases 97 and 104. It can be said that nonparoxysmal AV junctional tachycardia and ventricular bigeminy are the most common cardiac arrhythmias encountered in digitalis intoxication.

CASE 131

A 74-year-old man was admitted to the CCU because of a heart attack. He was not taking any medication before admission.
1. What is the cardiac rhythm diagnosis?
2. What is the proper therapeutic approach?

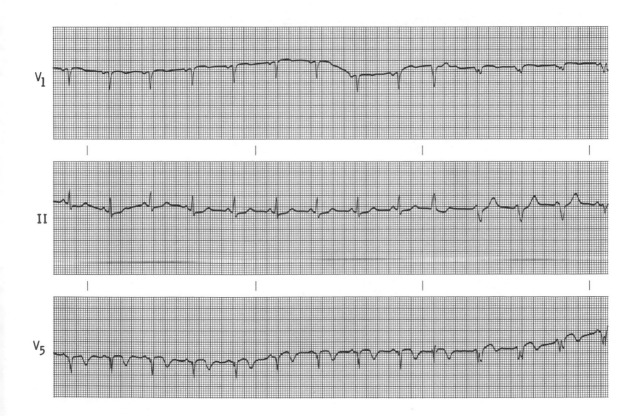

CASE 131: Diagnosis

The underlying cardiac rhythm is sinus (rate: 83 beats/min), but there are consecutively occurring bizarre beats initiated by a VPC at the end of this tracing. Nonparoxysmal ventricular tachycardia (accelerated ventricular rhythm or idioventricular tachycardia—rate: 80 beats/min) occurs independent of the sinus activity, causing AV dissociation. It is interesting to note that nonparoxysmal ventricular tachycardia is initiated by a VPC originating from another ectopic focus in the ventricles (the 10th beat).

Nonparoxysmal ventricular tachycardia is not uncommon during the first 24–72 hours of acute MI, but this arrhythmia is considered to be benign and self-limited. Thus, no treatment is necessary. In most cases, nonparoxysmal ventricular tachycardia occurs only transiently.

This patient suffered from extensive anterior MI.

CASE 132

This ECG tracing was obtained from an 80-year-old woman with known CAD. She was not taking any medication.
1. What is the cardiac rhythm diagnosis?
2. What is the proper therapeutic approach?

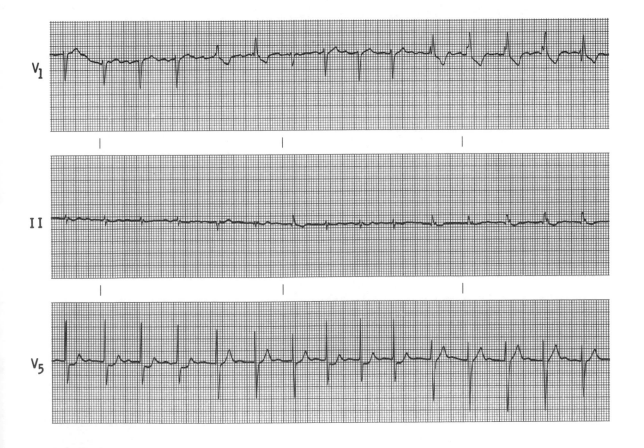

CASE 132: Diagnosis

The underlying cardiac rhythm is AF (rate: 95–110 beats/min), but bizarre beats occur intermittently with a regular ventricular cycle. Nonparoxysmal ventricular tachycardia (accelerated ventricular rhythm—rate: 95 beats/min) occurs independent of AF, leading to incomplete AV dissociation. Note that some QRS complexes show mixed configurations that represent ventricular fusion beats (e.g., the 5th, 6th, and 7th beats).

As discussed in Case 131, no treatment is indicated for nonparoxysmal ventricular tachycardia because of its benign nature.

CASE 133

Digitalis toxicity was suspected in a 71-year-old man who had suffered from extensive anterior MI 4 months previously.
1. What is the cardiac rhythm diagnosis?
2. What is the proper therapeutic approach?

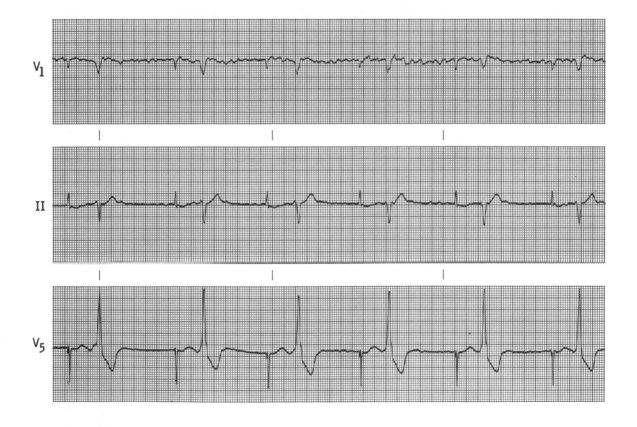

CASE 133: Diagnosis

The underlying cardiac rhythm is AF, but there are 2 types of QRS complexes with slow ventricular rate. The cardiac rhythm diagnosis is AF with advanced (high degree) AV block, causing intermittent AV junctional escape beats and frequent VPCs, producing ventricular bigeminy. The diagnosis of digitalis toxicity is almost certain when dealing with the arrhythmia shown in this ECG tracing.

The therapeutic approach to digitalis-induced arrhythmias has been discussed in Case 127.

The patient's 12-lead ECG shows evidences of extensive anterior MI (Q-S pattern in leads V_{1-6}—only V_1 and V_5 are shown here).

CASE 134

A 70-year-old man with severe CHF due to advanced chronic cor pulmonale and hyperthyroidism was admitted to the hospital because of intractable heart failure. He expired soon after this ECG tracing was taken.

1. What is the cardiac rhythm diagnosis?

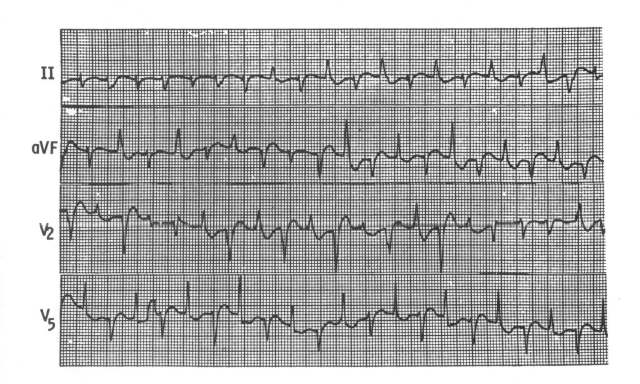

CASE 134: Diagnosis

Cardiac rhythm reveals AF with bidirectional ventricular tachycardia (ventricular rate: 165 beats/min), producing complete AV dissociation. His serum digoxin level was beyond 10 ng/ml, which is incompatible with life (therapeutic digoxin level: less than 2.5 ng/ml).

In bidirectional ventricular tachycardia, the atrial mechanism is nearly always ectopic rhythm, such as AF, atrial flutter, or atrial tachycardia. The underlying etiology for bidirectional ventricular tachycardia is almost always far-advanced digitalis toxicity, which is usually irreversible.

CASE 135

A 46-year-old man was admitted to the CCU because of acute anterior myocardial infarction. Soon after admission to the unit, he developed a very rapid heart action associated with hypotension and lightheadedness.

1. What is the cardiac rhythm diagnosis?
2. What is the treatment of choice?

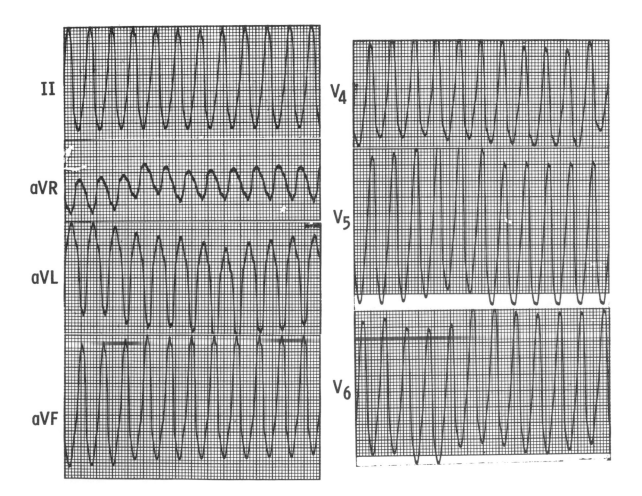

CASE 135: Diagnosis

The cardiac rhythm demonstrates a regular and rapid tachycardia (rate: 220 beats/min) with extremely bizarre QRS complexes. No P waves are discernible. In addition, a boundary between the QRS complex, S-T segment, and T wave is unclear, so that the entire complex appears to be a continuous loop form. Thus, the cardiac rhythm represents ventricular flutter, which has almost the same clinical significance as ventricular fibrillation. In fact, ventricular flutter soon leads to ventricular fibrillation and death unless the arrhythmia is terminated immediately.

The treatment of choice for ventricular flutter is immediate application of DC shock followed by intravenous infusion (2–4 mg/min) of lidocaine (Xylocaine) for at least 24–72 hours.

CASE 136

This ECG tracing was obtained from a 51-year-old man with acute anterior MI. Leads II-a, II-b, and II-c are not continuous.
1. What is the cardiac rhythm diagnosis?
2. What is the treatment of choice?

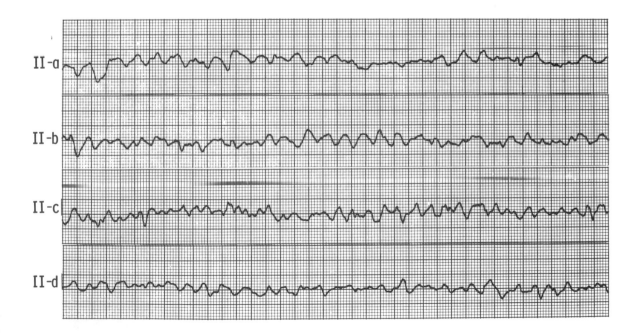

CASE 136: Diagnosis

This ECG tracing is a typical example of ventricular fibrillation, which consists of grossly irregular and chaotic ventricular rhythm.

The treatment of choice is DC shock with a defibrillator. Intravenous infusion (2–5 mg/min) of lidocaine is usually indicated following a termination of the arrhythmia in order to prevent recurrence of ventricular fibrillation.

CASE 137

These ECG rhythm strips were recorded on a 64-year-old man with cardiomyopathy, and he expired soon after this tracing was taken.
1. What is the cardiac rhythm diagnosis?
2. What is the proper therapeutic approach?

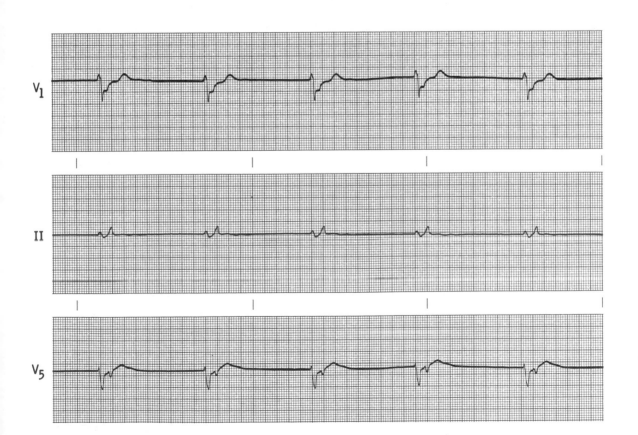

V₁

II

V₅

CASE 137: Diagnosis

It is obvious that the ventricular rate is extremely slow (rate: 33 beats/min) and the QRS complexes are broad and bizarre. The cardiac rhythm diagnosis is ventricular escape (idioventricular) rhythm with a rate of 33 beats/min. Note that each QRS complex is followed by a retrograde P wave (atrial capture).

Temporary artificial cardiac pacing with all available cardiopulmonary resuscitative measures should be applied immediately. Since this arrhythmia usually occurs in terminal cardiac illness in most cases, the prognosis is extremely grave.

Chapter 7
Differential Diagnosis of
Cardiac Arrhythmias

CASE 138

This ECG tracing was obtained from a 62-year-old man with long-standing COPD. He was not taking any cardiac drug.
1. What is the cardiac rhythm diagnosis?
2. What is the proper therapeutic approach?

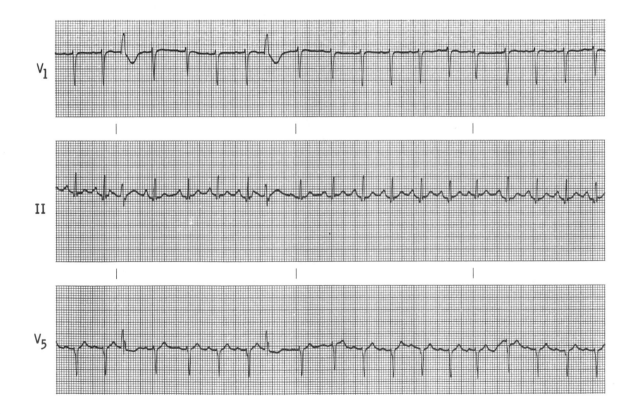

CASE 138: *Diagnosis*

The underlying cardiac rhythm is sinus tachycardia with a rate of 120 beats/min. Note that there are 3 ectopic beats, and 2 of them show bizarre QRS complexes (the 3rd and the 8th beats). All of these ectopic beats are APCs, and the first 2 APCs exhibit aberrant ventricular conduction (the 3rd and the 8th beats) as a result of very short coupling intervals. In addition, the P-R intervals of these APCs are markedly prolonged, again because of a very short coupling interval. The third APC (the 15th beat) originating from another focus shows normal QRS configuration because the coupling interval is not short.

An interesting finding in this ECG tracing is alteration of the P wave configuration of the sinus beat (the 4th and the 9th beats) immediately following APCs. This finding has been termed "aberrant atrial conduction" (Chung's phenomenon). Aberrant atrial conduction is considered to occur as a result of alteration of the refractory period in the atria following an APC. On rare occasions, aberrant atrial conduction may be observed following an AV junctional premature beat, a VPC, and parasystole (any origin).

No treatment is necessary for APCs. Aberrant atrial conduction is insignificant clinically.

CASE 139

An 81-year-old man was evaluated at the cardiac clinic because of his cardiac arrhythmia. He was not taking any medication.
1. What is the cardiac rhythm diagnosis?
2. What is the proper therapeutic approach?

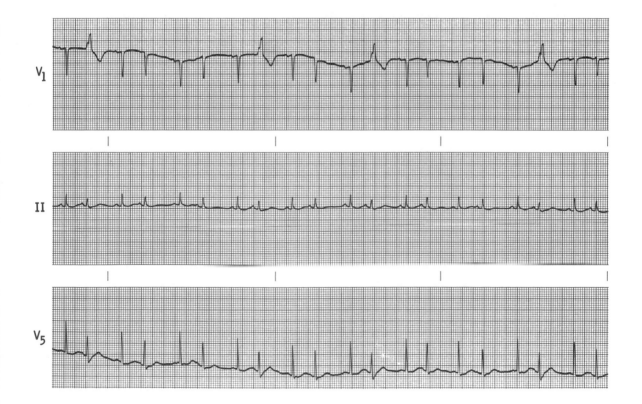

V_1

II

V_5

CASE 139: Diagnosis

The underlying cardiac rhythm is sinus tachycardia (rate: 116 beats/min), but there are frequent atrial ectopic beats causing atrial bigeminy. On superficial examination, there appear to be frequent APCs. When this arrhythmia is carefully studied, however, experienced readers should be able to appreciate that the coupling intervals vary and the interectopic intervals remain constant. Consequently, the diagnosis of atrial parasystole can be entertained. Note that many parasystolic beats exhibit bizarre QRS complexes as a result of aberrant ventricular conduction of different degree.

Parasystole is diagnosed when the coupling intervals vary and the shortest interectopic intervals are constant. When there is an exit block, the long interectopic interval shows a multiple of the shortest interectopic interval.

Clinically, parasystole is considered to be a benign cardiac arrhythmia. Thus, no treatment is necessary.

CASE 140

This ECG tracing was obtained from a 79-year-old man with slight hypertension. He was not taking any medication.
1. What is the cardiac rhythm diagnosis?
2. What is the ECG diagnosis?

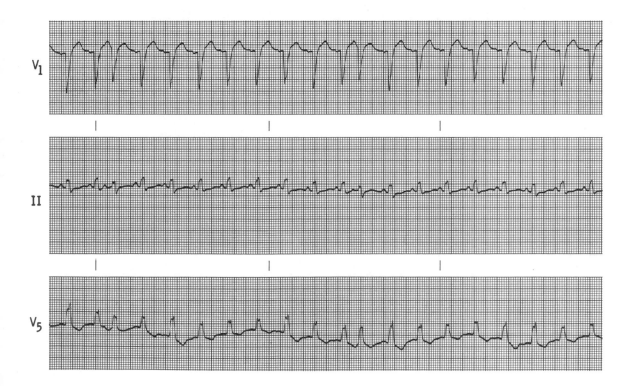

CASE 140: Diagnosis

The cardiac rhythm is sinus tachycardia with a rate of 120 beats/min. There are 2 APCs (the 3rd and 12th beats) that show slightly deformed QRS configurations as a result of aberrant ventricular conduction. Aberrant ventricular conduction occurs because the coupling interval is so short that the atrial premature impulse is conducted to the ventricles during their partial refractory period.

The diagnosis of LBBB is obvious to all readers. The broad and bizarre QRS configuration in APCs is due to 2 reasons, the preexisting LBBB and the aberrant ventricular conduction.

CASE 141

Cardiac consultation was requested on a 51-year-old woman with COPD for the evaluation of her cardiac arrhythmia. She was not taking any cardiac medication.
1. What is the cardiac rhythm diagnosis?
2. What is the proper therapeutic approach?

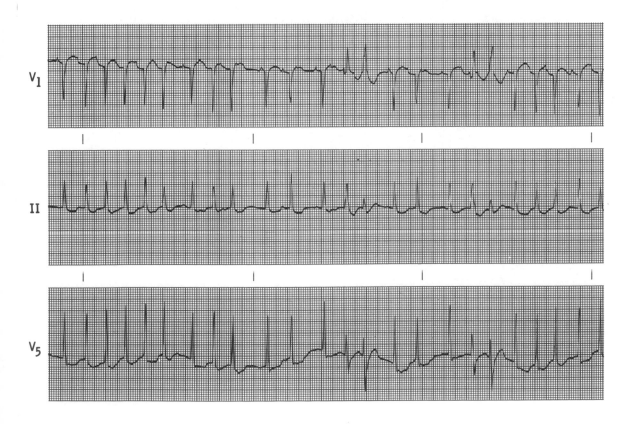

CASE 141: Diagnosis

On superficial examination, the cardiac rhythm appears to be AF because the cardiac cycle is grossly irregular and there are no clear P waves. However, experienced readers should be able to appreciate the rapidly occurring P waves of varying configurations. In addition, the P-P cycles vary with varying P-R intervals. Thus, the diagnosis of MAT can be entertained (atrail rate: 175 beats/min). There are 4 bizarre QRS complexes representing aberrant ventricular conduction as a result of Ashman's phenomenon.

Ashman's phenomenon is a physiologic phenomenon that is most commonly responsible for the production of aberrant ventricular conduction. The refractory period of the heart is directly influenced by the preceding cardiac cycle. The longer the R-R interval preceding a given cardiac cycle, the longer the refractory period following it; the shorter the R-R interval preceding a given cardiac cycle, the shorter is the refractory period following it. Ashman's phenomenon may be observed regardless of the underlying cardiac rhythm.

In this ECG tracing, the aberrantly conducted beats closely simulate VPCs. The most important therapeutic approach to MAT is the proper treatment of the underlying pulmonary disease (e.g., COPD). The efficacy of digitalis and various antiarrhythmic agents for MAT is often disappointing. MAT has been described in Case 68. It has been shown that COPD is the most common underlying disorder responsible for the production of MAT.

The diagnosis of left ventricular hypertrophy can be made without any difficulty.

CASE 142

A 62-year-old man was admitted to the intermediate CCU because of acute CHF associated with rapid heart rate. He was not taking any medication before admission.

1. What is the cardiac rhythm diagnosis?
2. What is the proper therapeutic approach?

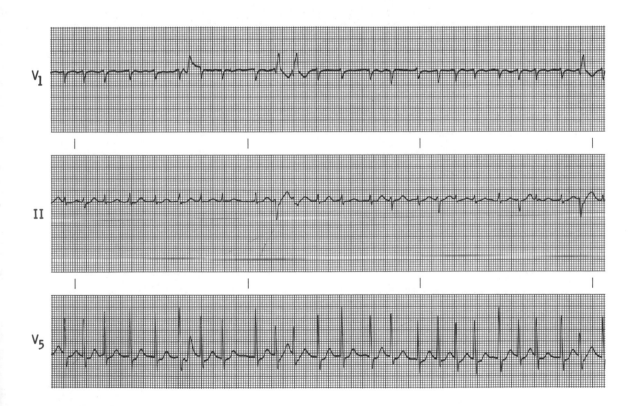

CASE 142: Diagnosis

The cardiac rhythm is AF with rapid ventricular response (rate: 140–165 beats/min). Some QRS complexes are bizarre because of aberrant ventricular conduction. The aberrantly conducted beats resemble VPCs, but a lack of any pause following a bizarre beat excludes the possibility of VPC. Ashman's phenomenon is clearly the cause of the aberrant ventricular conduction in some areas (the 10th and 11th beats). Otherwise, a very short cardiac cycle (rapid rate) is responsible for the production of aberrant ventricular conduction.

Aberrant ventricular conduction is most commonly (80–85%) manifested by RBBB pattern as seen in this tracing. LBBB pattern or hemiblock pattern is only occasionally observed during aberrant ventricular conduction. Rarely, a combination of RBBB and left anterior hemiblock pattern may be observed during aberrant ventricular conduction.

The treatment of choice for AF with rapid ventricular response is rapid digitalization. If the clinical situation is extremely urgent, however, DC shock should be applied immediately.

CASE 143

This ECG tracing was taken on a 65-year-old man. He was not taking any medication.
1. What is the cardiac rhythm diagnosis?
2. What is the proper therapeutic approach?

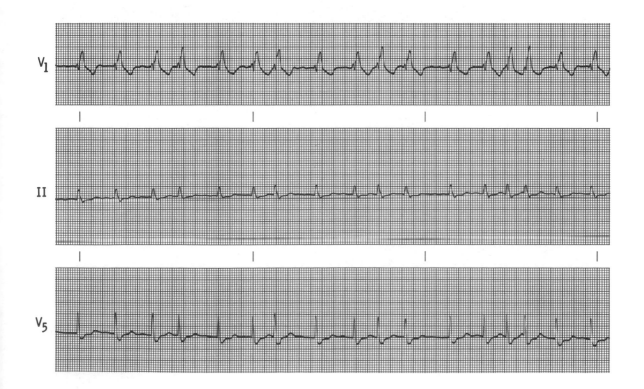

CASE 143: Diagnosis

The cardiac rhythm is AF with moderately rapid ventricular response (rate: 100–130 beats/min). The QRS complexes are broad and bizarre because of RBBB. Consequently, AF with RBBB superficially mimics ventricular tachycardia.

The proper therapeutic approach is moderately rapid digitalization.

CASE 144

A 55-year-old woman was examined at a cardiologist's office because of palpitations. She was not taking any medication.
1. What is the cardiac rhythm diagnosis?
2. What is the proper therapeutic approach?

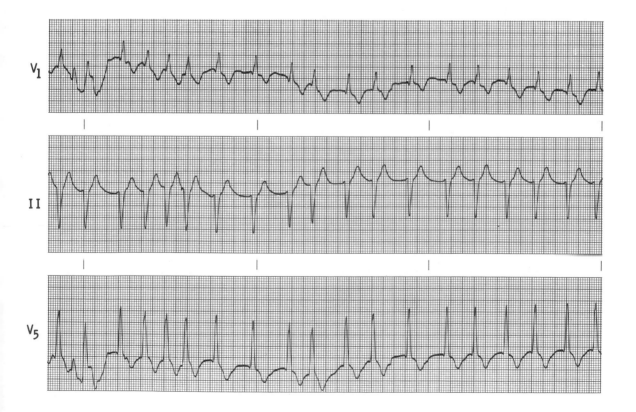

CASE 144: *Diagnosis*

The cardiac rhythm is AF with moderately rapid ventricular response (rate: 120–155 beats/min). The QRS complexes are broad and bizarre because of the preexisting BFB consisting of RBBB and left anterior hemiblock. Ventricular tachycardia is superficially simulated.

The treatment of choice is moderately rapid digitalization. Artificial cardiac pacing is not indicated for chronic asymptomatic BFB.

CASE 145

This ECG tracing of a 77-year-old woman was presented at a weekly cardiology conference because of the interesting ECG finding.
1. What is the ECG diagnosis?

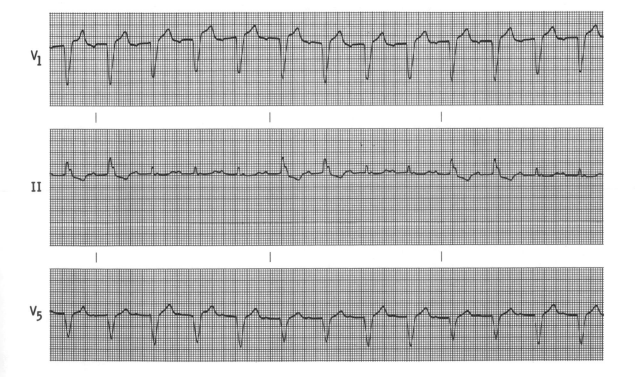

CASE 145: Diagnosis

The cardiac rhythm is sinus (rate: 80 beats/min) with first degree AV block (P-R interval: 0.28 second). There are 2 kinds of QRS complexes because complete and incomplete LBBB occurs intermittently unrelated to the heart rate. Of course, this ECG finding is insignificant clinically.

CASE 146

This ECG tracing was obtained from a 68-year-old woman who complained of palpitations. She was not taking any medication.
1. What is the cardiac rhythm diagnosis?
2. What is the proper therapeutic approach?

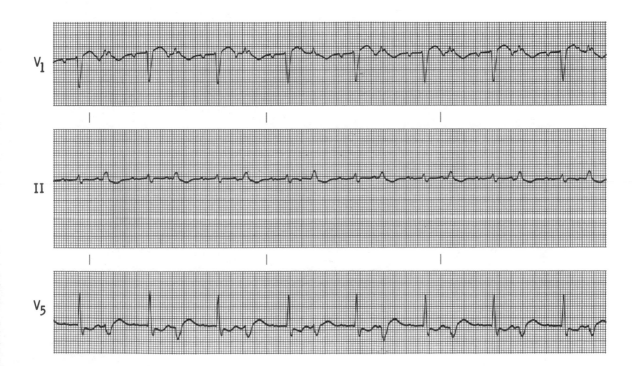

CASE 146: *Diagnosis*

The underlying cardiac rhythm is sinus tachycardia with a rate of 104 beats/min and first degree AV block. Note the frequent VPCs that occur on every other beat, leading to ventricular bigeminy. The VPCs are considered to be originating from the left ventricle, judging from the upright QRS complex in lead V_1 and the negative QRS complex in lead V_5.

Since the VPCs cause significant symptoms (i.e., palpitations), the arrhythmia requires treatment. Any predisposing factor, such as excessive consumption of coffee, should be eliminated (see Case 119). Otherwise, a proper antiarrhythmic agent (e.g., quinidine, propranolol) should be given (see Cases 117 and 119).

Left atrial hypertrophy and intraventricular block (diffuse or nonspecific) are diagnosed.

CASE 147

These ECG rhythm strips were taken on a 73-year-old woman soon after coronary artery bypass surgery. Her hemodynamic and clinical status was said to be satisfactory.
1. What is the cardiac rhythm diagnosis?
2. What is the proper therapeutic approach?

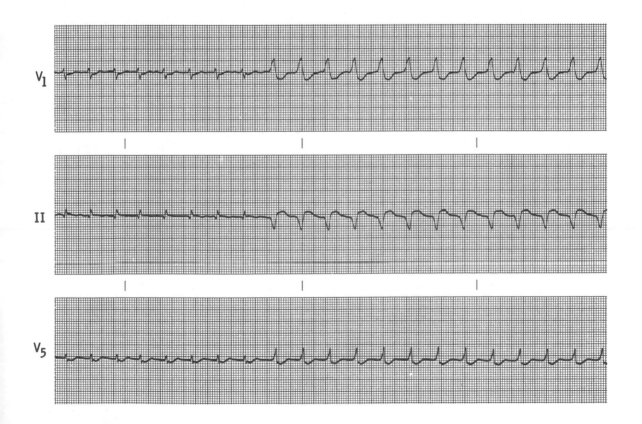

V₁

II

V₅

CASE 147: *Diagnosis*

It is obvious that there are 2 kinds of QRS complexes. No P waves are discernible. The cardiac rhythm diagnosis is nonparoxysmal AV junctional tachycardia (rate: 140 beats/min) followed by nonparoxysmal ventricular tachycardia (rate: 130 beats/min).

Both nonparoxysmal AV junctional tachycardia and nonparoxysmal ventricular tachycardia are not uncommon soon after any major cardiac surgery. These arrhythmias are considered to be benign and self-limited. Thus, no active treatment is necessary.

CASE 148

Digitalis toxicity was suspected in a 60-year-old woman.
1. What is the cardiac rhythm diagnosis?
2. What is the proper therapeutic approach?

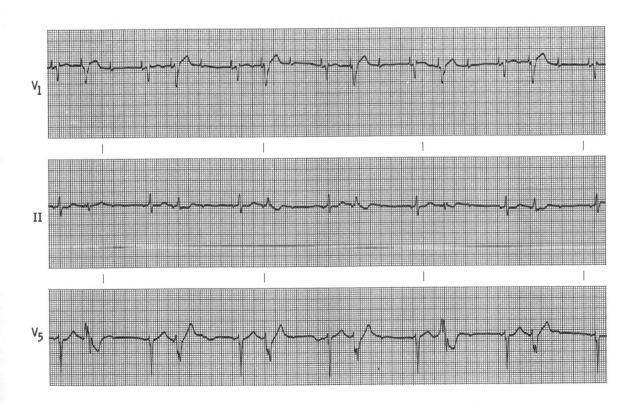

V₁

II

V₅

CASE 148: Diagnosis

The cardiac rhythm is nonparoxysmal AV junctional tachycardia (rate: 110 beats/min) with 3:1 AV block and frequent VPCs, causing ventricular bigeminy.

As repeatedly emphasized (see Cases 97 and 104), nonparoxysmal AV junctional tachycardia and ventricular bigeminy are the most common digitalis-induced cardiac arrhythmias. The therapeutic approach to digitalis-induced cardiac arrhythmias has been described in Case 104.

CASE 149

A 50-year-old woman developed a rapid heart action suddenly during an emotional upset. She was not taking any medication.
1. What is the cardiac rhythm diagnosis?
2. What is the proper therapeutic approach?

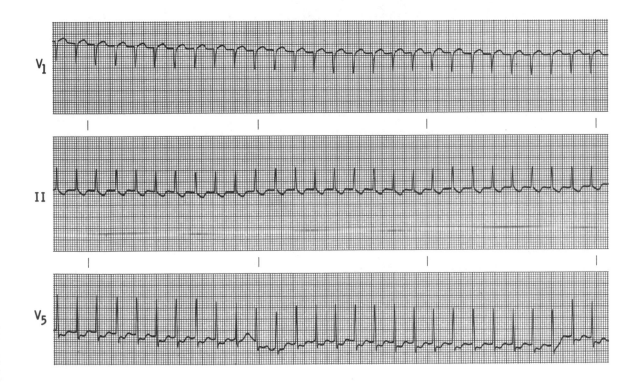

CASE 149: Diagnosis

The cardiac rhythm diagnosis is supraventricular tachycardia with a rate of 175 beats/min. Note that the cardiac cycle is regular and the QRS complexes are normal with no discernible P waves. Under this circumstance, the term "supraventricular tachycardia" can be used without specifying the exact origin of the tachycardia. In reality, however, supraventricular tachycardia may be paroxysmal atrial or AV junctional tachycardia or reciprocating tachycardia. In any case, a re-entry mechanism in the AV junction is considered to be responsible.

The proper diagnostic and therapeutic approaches to supraventricular tachycardia have been described previously (see Case 67). CSS is often effective in terminating supraventricular tachycardia. Otherwise, propranolol is considered to be the agent of choice in most such cases.

CASE 150

This ECG tracing was obtained from a 51-year-old woman with COPD.
1. What is the cardiac rhythm diagnosis?
2. What is the proper therapeutic approach?

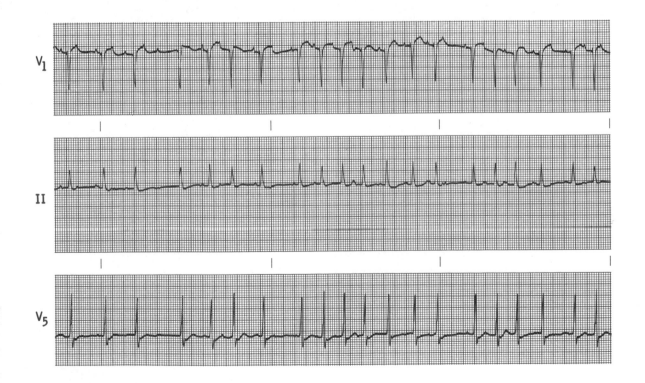

V₁

II

V₅

CASE 150: Diagnosis

The cardiac rhythm is MAT with a rate of 175 beats/min and varying degree AV block. Note that the P-P intervals as well as P-R intervals vary and the P wave configurations also vary. Some P waves are not conducted to the ventricles (a common feature of MAT).

The most important therapeutic approach to MAT is aggressive treatment of the underlying pulmonary disease. MAT has been described in detail in Case 68.

CASE 151

This ECG tracing was obtained from a 75-year-old woman several hours after cholecystectomy. Pulmonary embolism was suspected.
1. What is the cardiac rhythm diagnosis?
2. What is the proper therapeutic approach?
3. What ECG abnormalities are commonly caused by pulmonary embolism?

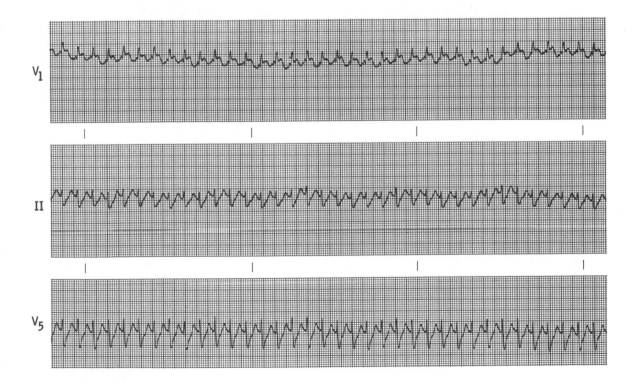

CASE 151: Diagnosis

The cardiac rhythm diagnosis is supraventricular tachycardia (rate: 225 beats/min), which may be atrial tachycardia or flutter with 1:1 AV conduction. Incomplete RBBB is diagnosed without any difficulty.

The therapeutic approach to supraventricular tachycardia has been described in Case 67. Most often, CSS is the first therapeutic step. If the procedure is ineffective, various postoperative tachyarrhythmias are best treated with beta-blocking agents, such as propranolol. If the clinical situation is extremely urgent, DC shock should be applied immediately.

Pulmonary embolism may produce a variety of ECG findings, but these ECG abnormalities are often transient. Various ECG abnormalities caused by pulmonary embolism may include:

1. Sinus tachycardia
2. Various supraventricular tachyarrhythmias (e.g., AF)
3. RBBB (complete or incomplete)
4. Right axis deviation with or without posterior axis deviation of the QRS complexes
5. P-pulmonale
6. S_1-Q_3 pattern (rare)
7. $S_1-S_2-S_3$ pattern (rare)
8. Left axis deviation (extremely rare)
9. Pseudodiaphragmatic MI

CASE 152

A 73-year-old man was brought to the emergency room because of his rapid heart action. He had recovered from a heart attack that occurred 3 months previously. He was not taking any medication.
1. What is the cardiac rhythm diagnosis?
2. What is the proper therapeutic approach?

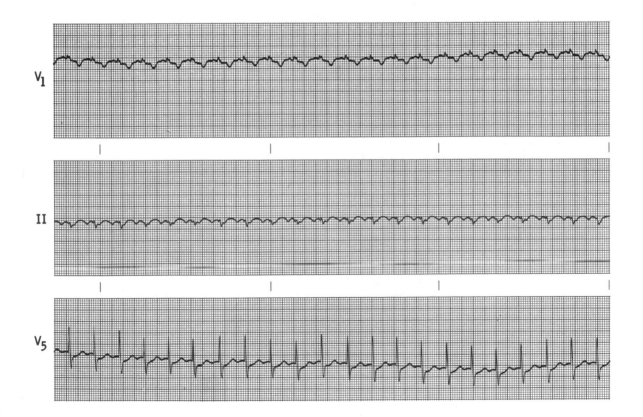

CASE 152: Diagnosis

The cardiac rhythm is atrial flutter (atrial rate: 270 beats/min) with 2:1 AV conduction (ventricular rate: 135 beats/min). The ventricular cycle is precisely regular, and every other flutter wave is conducted to the ventricles. The diagnosis of atrial flutter with 2:1 AV conduction is a strong possibility when the ventricular cycle is regular, with ventricular rate ranging from 125 to 175 beats/min.

The diagnostic and therapeutic approaches to atrial flutter with 2:1 AV conduction have been described in Cases 81 and 83.

The diagnosis of incomplete RBBB can be made without any difficulty.

CASE 153

This ECG tracing was obtained from a 51-year-old woman with rheumatic heart disease. Her medications included digoxin 0.25 mg once and quinidine 0.3 g 4 times daily.
1. What is the cardiac rhythm diagnosis?

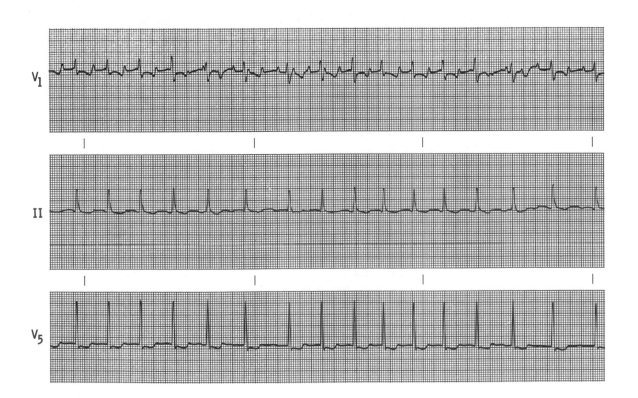

CASE 153: Diagnosis

The cardiac rhythm is atrial flutter (atrial rate: 230 beats/min) with varying AV response. The atrial flutter cycle is slower than usual (the usual flutter cycle ranging from 250 to 350 beats/min) because of the quinidine effect.

Her 12-lead ECG shows biventricular hypertrophy (not shown here). Biventricular hypertrophy is diagnosed on the basis of right axis deviation, relatively tall R waves in leads V_{1-2}, and tall R waves in leads V_{5-6} (diagnostic of left ventricular hypertrophy).

CASE 154

A 67-year-old man was examined at the cardiac clinic as a follow-up medical checkup.

1. What is the cardiac rhythm diagnosis?

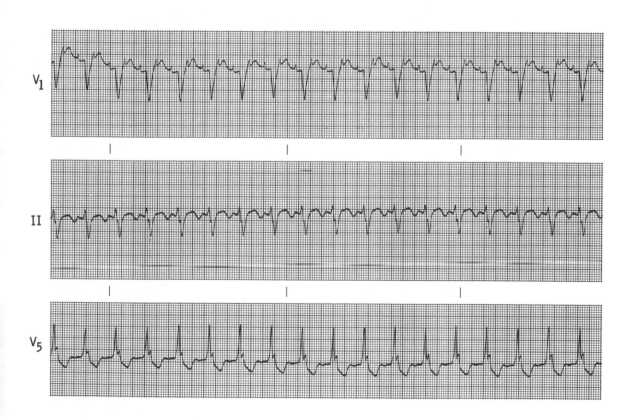

CASE 154: *Diagnosis*

On superficial examination, the cardiac rhythm appears to be non-paroxysmal AV junctional tachycardia because the P waves seem to be inverted in lead II. However, the correct rhythm diagnosis is atrial flutter (atrial rate: 240 beats/min) with 2:1 AV conduction. The flutter waves are clearly shown in lead V_1. The atrial flutter cycle is slower than usual secondary due to the quinidine effect.

The diagnosis of LBBB can be established without any difficulty.

CASE 155

This ECG tracing was taken on a 66-year-old man. His only medication was quinidine 0.3 g 4 times daily by mouth.
1. What is the cardiac rhythm diagnosis?

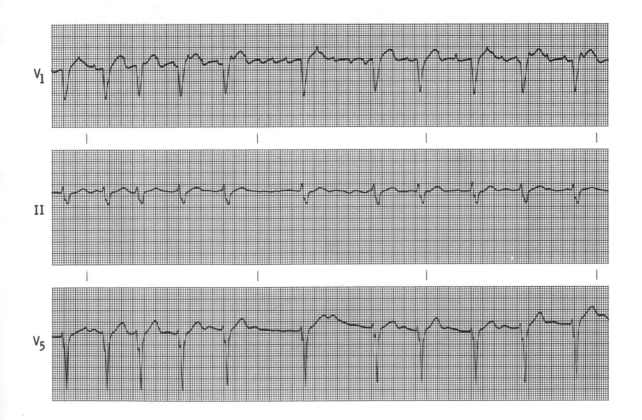

CASE 155: Diagnosis

The cardiac rhythm is atrial flutter (atrial rate: 220–280 beats/min) with varying degree advanced AV block. An interesting ECG finding in this tracing is markedly irregular atrial flutter cycle with varying configurations of the flutter waves. These findings are most commonly due to quinidine or quinidinelike drugs (e.g., procainamide). Otherwise, irregular flutter cycles may be observed in patients with cardiomyopathy.

The diagnosis of LBBB is suggested.

CASE 156

Cardiac consultation was requested on a 74-year-old man because his cardiac rhythm was considered to be somewhat unusual.

1. What is the cardiac rhythm diagnosis?

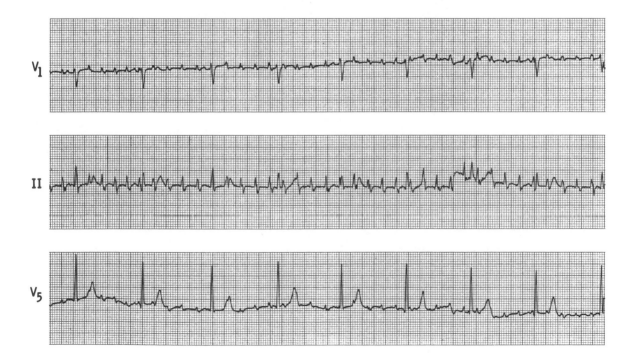

CASE 156: Diagnosis

The patient's cardiac rhythm appears to be atrial flutter with complete AV block, producing AV junctional escape rhythm. However, experienced readers should be able to recognize that these rapidly occurring waves are artifacts due to extracardiac muscle tremors. Thus, the actual cardiac rhythm is sinus bradycardia with a rate of 53 beats/min.

This patient was found to have Parkinson's disease. When all artifacts are abolished after medication, his sinus bradycardia is confirmed (not shown here).

CASE 157

Aortic valve replacement was performed on a 48-year-old man with aortic stenosis. Before surgery, his ECG revealed normal sinus rhythm with LBBB.

1. What is the cardiac rhythm diagnosis?
2. What is the proper therapeutic approach?

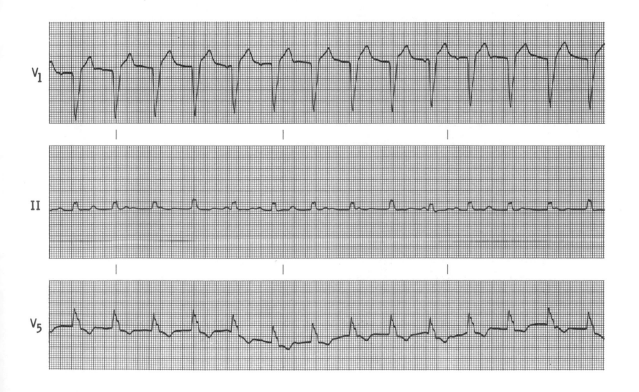

CASE 157: Diagnosis

The cardiac rhythm is sinus tachycardia (atrial rate: 102 beats/min) with nonparoxysmal AV junctional tachycardia (ventricular rate: 85 beats/min), producing complete AV dissociation. Most readers should be able to recognize regularly occurring sinus P waves, which are independent of the QRS complexes (meaning AV dissociation).

Nonparoxysmal AV junctional tachycardia is not uncommonly observed immediately after various cardiac operations, but this arrhythmia is found to be self-limited and usually transient. Thus, no treatment is necessary under this circumstance.

LBBB is very common in patients with long-standing and severe aortic stenosis.

CASE 158

This ECG tracing was taken soon after mitral valve replacement for rheumatic mitral stenosis.
1. What is the cardiac rhythm diagnosis?
2. What is the proper therapeutic approach?

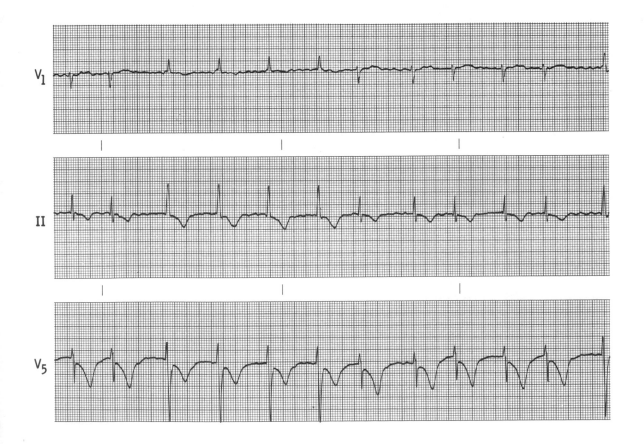

CASE 158: Diagnosis

The underlying cardiac rhythm is AF, but bizarre QRS complexes occur intermittently. These bizarre beats are considered to be originating from one of the fascicles of the left bundle branch system. Thus, the cardiac rhythm diagnosis is AF with intermittent fascicular tachycardia (rate: 72 beats/min), producing incomplete AV dissociation. The fascicular beat is only slightly bizarre and relatively narrow, but, in a broad sense, the fascicular tachycardia belongs to ventricular tachycardia.

Fascicular tachycardia is not uncommon during the immediate postoperative period following any cardiac surgery. No treatment is necessary, however, because fascicular tachycardia is benign and self-limited.

Diffuse T wave inversion is compatible with the postcardiotomy syndrome.

CASE 159

A 66-year-old woman developed a very rapid heart action soon after admission to the CCU with the diagnosis of acute anterior MI.
1. What is the cardiac rhythm diagnosis?
2. What is the proper therapeutic approach?

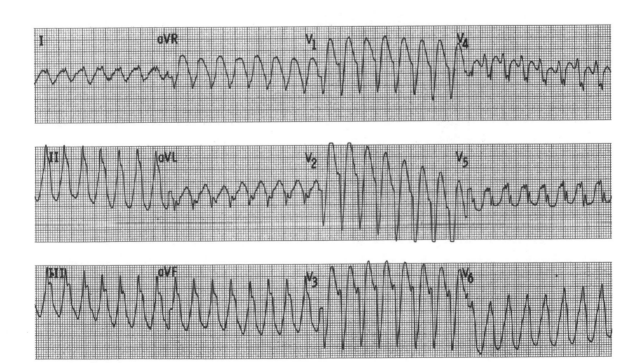

CASE 159: Diagnosis

The cardiac rhythm is paroxysmal ventricular tachycardia with a rate of 196 beats/min. This arrhythmia may be termed "preflutter" ventricular tachycardia because the boundary between the QRS complex, the S-T segment, and the T wave is ill-defined, and the entire ECG complex appears to be a continuous loop.

The best therapeutic approach to paroxysmal ventricular tachycardia with very rapid rate or ventricular flutter is immediate application of DC shock. Following the termination of ventricular tachycardia, ventricular flutter, or ventricular fibrillation by DC shock, continuous intravenous infusion of lidocaine is highly recommended for at least 24–72 hours.

CASE 160

A 43-year-old, apparently healthy woman was referred to a cardiologist for evaluation of her arrhythmia. She had no complaint and was not taking any medication. The cardiac rhythm strips (tracing A) and her 12-lead ECG (tracing B) were recorded consecutively on the same day.

1. What is the cardiac rhythm diagnosis?
2. What is the proper therapeutic approach?

A

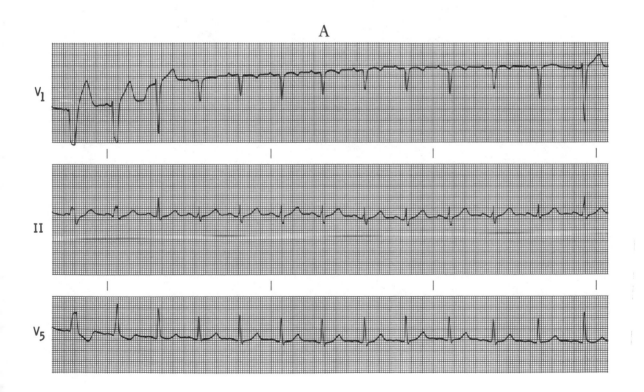

CASE 160: Diagnosis

The underlying cardiac rhythm is sinus with a rate of 78 beats/min, but some QRS complexes are broad and bizarre. Experienced readers should be able to appreciate that all broad QRS complexes occur independently of the atrial activity. Thus, the correct rhythm diagnosis is sinus rhythm with intermittent nonparoxysmal ventricular tachycardia (rate: 75 beats/min), producing incomplete AV dissociation.

There are frequent ventricular fusion beats, which superficially resemble intermittent WPW syndrome. Otherwise, intermittent LBBB is superficially simulated.

It has been shown that nonparoxysmal ventricular tachycardia is clinically benign and self-limited. Accordingly, no treatment is indicated. Although nonparoxysmal ventricular tachycardia is most commonly observed during the first 72 hours of acute MI, this arrhythmia may occasionally occur in healthy people.

B

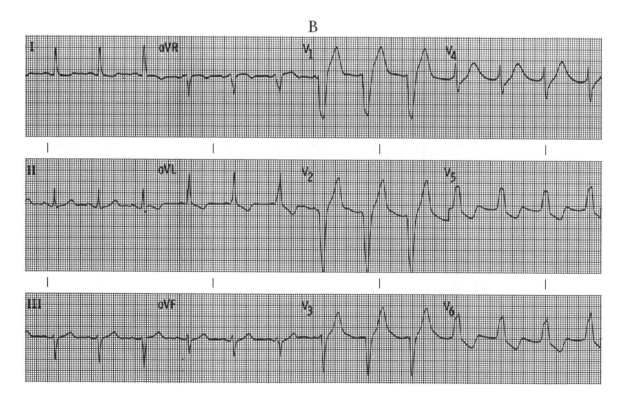

Chapter 8
Wolff-Parkinson-White Syndrome

CASE 161

This ECG tracing was obtained from a 29-year-old man as a part of preoperative (noncardiac) evaluation.
1. What is the ECG diagnosis?
2. What is the proper therapeutic approach?

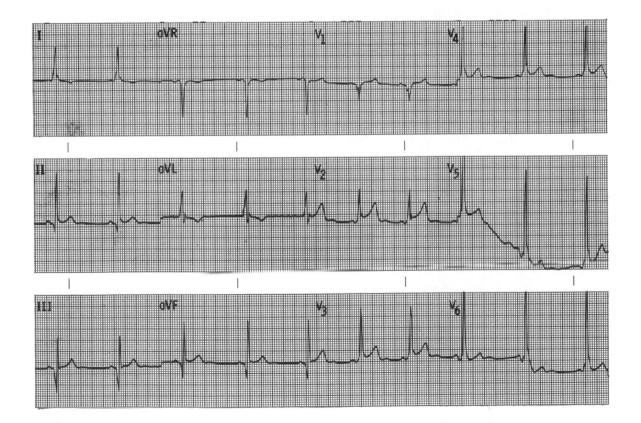

CASE 161: Diagnosis

The cardiac rhythm is sinus bradycardia and arrhythmia with rates ranging from 52 to 63 beats/min.

Experienced readers should be able to diagnose WPW syndrome, type B, without much difficulty.

The diagnostic criteria of WPW syndrome include a short P-R interval with a broad QRS complex due to a delta-wave. This unique ECG finding is considered to be due to a premature activation of a portion of the ventricles via an accessory pathway.

Type B WPW syndrome is diagnosed when the delta wave is directed posteriorly and to the left so that lead V_1 shows Q-S or rS wave, whereas leads V_{5-6} reveal positive (upright) QRS complexes, as shown in this tracing. On the other hand, the delta-wave is directed anteriorly and to the right in type A WPW syndrome so that a tall or relatively tall R wave is shown in lead V_1 (often up to leads V_{2-3}) and Q-S waves or Q-R waves in leads V_{5-6} (see Cases 162, 165, 166, and 167).

In both types A and B WPW syndrome, delta-waves are directed superiorly in many cases, so that a pseudodiaphragmatic MI pattern is produced, as seen in this ECG tracing.

It is well documented that various supraventricular tachyarrhythmias are frequently associated with WPW syndrome (see Cases 169 and 170). However, no treatment is necessary as long as the individual is free of documented tachyarrhythmias associated with the WPW syndrome.

High left ventricular voltage is very common among healthy young people. Thus, this ECG finding is a normal variant (not left ventricular hypertrophy).

CASE 162

A 31-year-old man was referred to a cardiac clinic for the evaluation of his frequent episodes of palpitations. He was not taking any medication.
1. What is the ECG diagnosis?
2. What is the proper therapeutic approach?

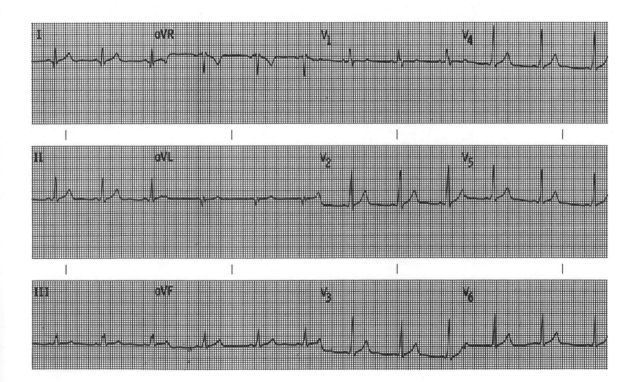

CASE 162: Diagnosis

The cardiac rhythm is sinus with a rate of 68 beats/min. WPW syndrome, type A, can be diagnosed without much difficulty (see Case 161).

For the diagnostic step to document any transient tachyarrhythmia, the Holter monitor ECG should be obtained. If necessary, the Holter monitor ECG should be repeated until any expected tachyarrhythmia is recorded.

When the Holter monitor ECG fails to record any tachyarrhythmia, an electrophysiologic study should be carried out in individuals with significant symptoms (e.g., palpitations) associated with WPW syndrome. It is possible to induce various tachyarrhythmias by a variety of electrophysiologic techniques. In addition, the best effective antiarrhythmic agent can be selected for a given tachyarrhythmia also by electrophysiologic study.

In addition to WPW syndrome, incomplete RBBB is diagnosed.

CASE 163

This ECG tracing was taken on a 20-year-old, apparently healthy man. He was not taking any medication.

1. What is the ECG diagnosis?

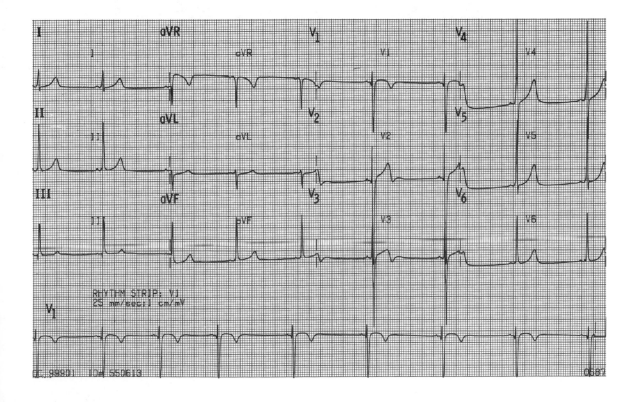

CASE 163: Diagnosis

The cardiac rhythm is sinus bradycardia and sinus arrhythmia with rates ranging from 45 to 56 beats/min.

Inexperienced readers may not recognize delta-waves in this ECG tracing because the duration of the delta-wave is very minimal. However, experienced readers should be able to diagnose WPW syndrome, type B. Some investigators use the term "Lown-Ganong-Levine (LGL) syndrome" when the delta-wave is so minimal that the ECG tracing reveals a normal (narrow) or near-normal QRS complex with a short P-R interval associated with tachyarrhythmias. The LGL syndrome is considered to be a variant of the WPW syndrome.

In addition, the diagnosis of "juvenile T wave pattern" is made on the basis of biphasic to inverted T waves in leads V_{1-3}. However, the juvenile T wave pattern is a normal variant, common in healthy young individuals. High left ventricular voltage is also a common finding in healthy young people and is a normal variant.

CASE 164

This ECG tracing of a 36-year-old woman was presented at the weekly ECG conference because the ECG finding was considered to be somewhat unusual.

1. What is the ECG diagnosis?

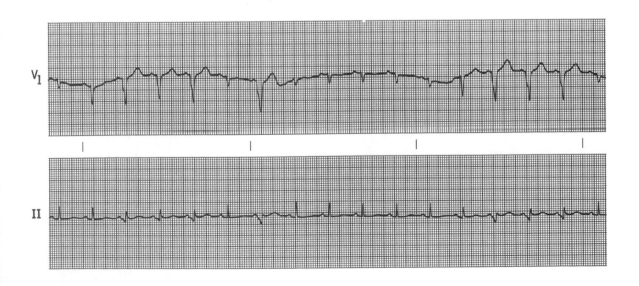

CASE 164: *Diagnosis*

The cardiac rhythm is sinus with a rate of 98 beats/min. It is obvious that there are 2 kinds of QRS complexes. This ECG finding represents intermittent WPW syndrome, type B. It is interesting to note that some QRS complexes reveal an intermediate form, which is due to a ventricular fusion beat. Ventricular fusion beats occur when the cardiac impulses are conducted to the ventricles simultaneously via the normal AV conduction system and an accessory pathway.

CASE 165

A 31-year-old woman was seen at the cardiac clinic for the first time
because of frequent episodes of palpitations since her early childhood.
She was not taking any medication, however.
1. What is the ECG diagnosis?
2. What is the proper therapeutic approach?

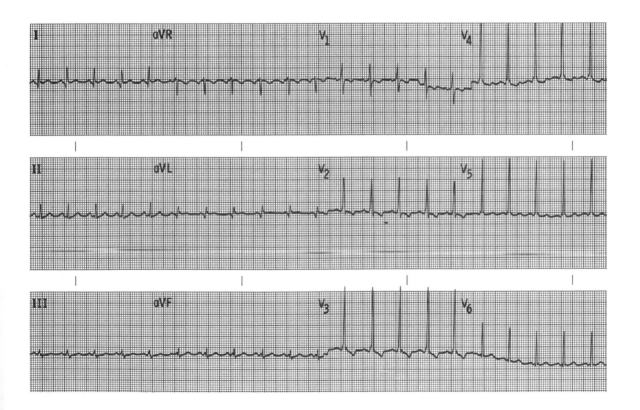

CASE 165: Diagnosis

The cardiac rhythm is sinus tachycardia with a rate of 120 beats/min. At first glance, her ECG seems to be within normal limits because the delta-waves are not so obvious in every lead. However, experienced readers should be able to diagnose WPW syndrome, type A, without much difficulty (see Case 161). The delta-waves are most obvious in leads V_{1-4}.

As emphasized in Case 161, it is essential to document the tachyarrhythmia so that a proper antiarrhythmic agent can be administered. Needless to say, the Holter monitor ECG is the most valuable tool to document any transient tachyarrhythmia. If the repeated Holter monitor ECGs fail to record the expected tachyarrhythmia, electrophysiologic study should strongly be considered.

CASE 166

A 24-year-old man was presented during the weekly professor round because of an interesting ECG finding. He was admitted to the medical service because of infectious mononucleosis, and the ECG abnormality shown in this tracing was an incidental finding.

1. What is the ECG diagnosis?

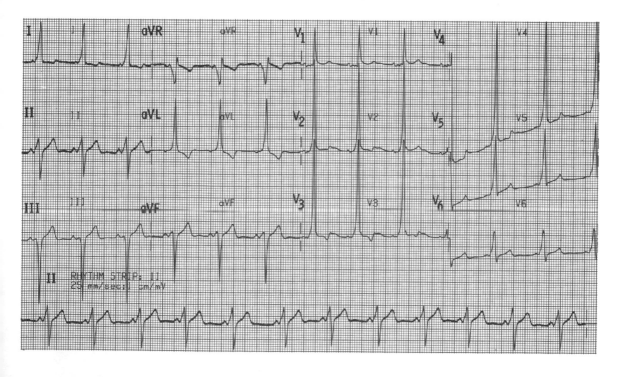

CASE 166: Diagnosis

The cardiac rhythm is sinus arrhythmia with a rate of 75 beats/min. Even inexperienced physicians should be able to diagnose WPW syndrome, type A, because the delta-waves are so obvious in all ECG leads. It should be noted that the P-R interval is short and the QRS complex is broad as a result of the delta-wave.

Another ECG abnormality is left anterior hemiblock (QRS axis: −45 degrees).

As emphasized repeatedly, the most important clinical significance of WPW syndrome is the frequent occurrence of various tachyarrhythmias (see Cases 169 and 170).

CASE 167

This ECG tracing was obtained from a 67-year-old man during his annual medical checkup. He had no complaint and was not taking any medication.

1. What is the ECG diagnosis?

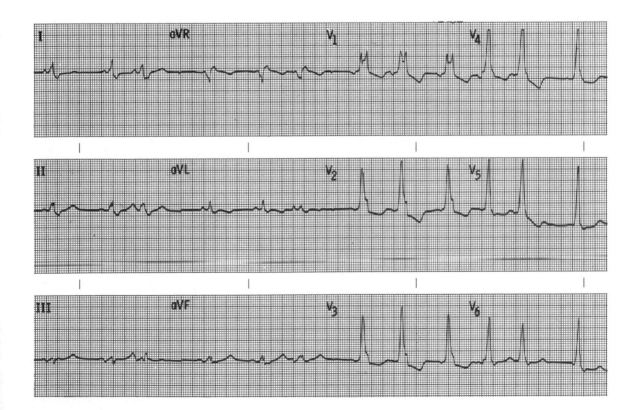

CASE 167: Diagnosis

The underlying cardiac rhythm is sinus bradycardia (rate: 56 beats/min), but there are frequent APCs. RBBB is easily recognized using conventional diagnostic criteria. Another coexisting ECG abnormality is possible WPW syndrome, type A, although a coexisting posterior MI is an alternative diagnostic possibility. Note that the first R wave of the RR′ in lead V_1 is much taller than expected because of the coexisting WPW syndrome, type A, or a posterior MI.

CASE 168

Cardiac consultation was requested on a 22-year-old man because a heart murmur was heard. A congenital heart disease was suspected.
1. What is the ECG diagnosis?
2. What congenital heart disease is most likely present judging from the ECG findings?

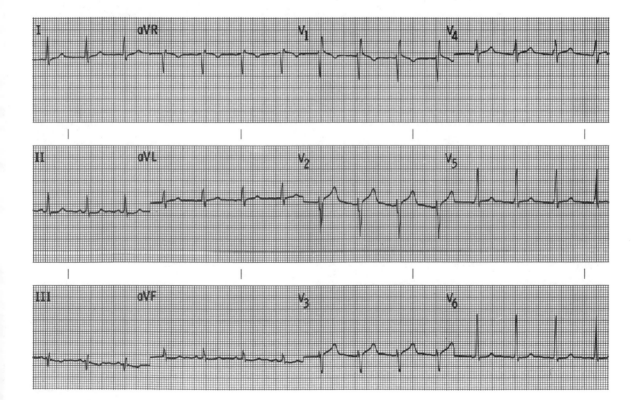

CASE 168: Diagnosis

The cardiac rhythm is sinus with a rate of 88 beats/min. The diagnosis of incomplete RBBB can be made without much difficulty. In addition, most experienced readers may be able to diagnose WPW syndrome, type B. The delta-waves are best shown in leads V_{4-6}.

As far as the underlying congenital heart disease is concerned, atrial septal defect is most commonly associated with RBBB (particularly the incomplete form). In a broad sense, WPW syndrome is also a form of congenital heart disease. Thus, this patient has 2 congenital cardiac diseases, atrial septal defect and WPW syndrome.

It has been shown that WPW syndrome is often associated with various congenital heart diseases, including atrial septal defect, mitral valve prolapse syndrome, and Ebstein's anomaly.

CASE 169

A 53-year-old man experienced many episodes of rapid heart actions, and this ECG tracing was taken during one of the episodes associated with palpitations. WPW syndrome was suspected.
1. What is the cardiac rhythm diagnosis?
2. What is the proper therapeutic approach?

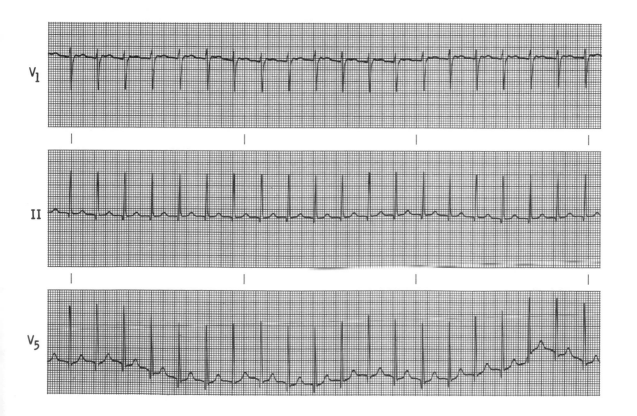

CASE 169: Diagnosis

The cardiac rhythm is supraventricular tachycardia with a rate of 130 beats/min. There are no visible P waves, and the ventricular cycle is regular with normal QRS complexes. Under this circumstance, the term "reciprocating tachycardia" or "reentrant tachycardia" is commonly used because the fundamental mechanism responsible for the production of the tachycardia is proven to be a reentry phenomenon.

In WPW syndrome, reciprocating tachycardia is the most common rapid heart action observed. AF or atrial flutter is much less common in WPW syndrome (see Case 170).

In reciprocating tachycardia in WPW syndrome, the QRS complexes are normal (narrow) in most cases, and broad QRS complexes as a result of anomalous AV conduction are uncommon. On the other hand, AF or atrial flutter is nearly always associated with anomalous AV conduction, causing broad QRS complexes (see Case 170).

Therapeutically, beta-blockers (e.g., propranolol) are found to be very effective for reciprocating tachycardia with normal QRS complexes in WPW syndrome. Digitalis or verapamil is the second drug of choice under this circumstance. When the QRS complexes are broad because of anomalous AV conduction in WPW syndrome (e.g., AF with anomalous AV conduction—see Case 170), intravenous injection of lidocaine is considered to be the treatment of choice. Quinidine or procainamide is almost equally effective under this circumstance.

Recently, it has been shown that amiodarone (still an investigative agent in the USA) is very effective in the treatment and prevention of all types of tachyarrhythmias associated with WPW syndrome, since amiodarone is capable of blocking the conduction in the normal AV conduction system as well as in the accessory pathway.

If the clinical situation is urgent, immediate application of DC shock is the treatment of choice for any type of tachyarrhythmia.

CASE 170

A 46-year-old man was brought to the emergency room because of a very rapid heart action with acute onset. He had had similar episodes on many occasions in the past but was not taking any medication on a regular basis.
1. What is the cardiac rhythm diagnosis?
2. What is the underlying disorder?
3. What is the proper therapeutic approach?

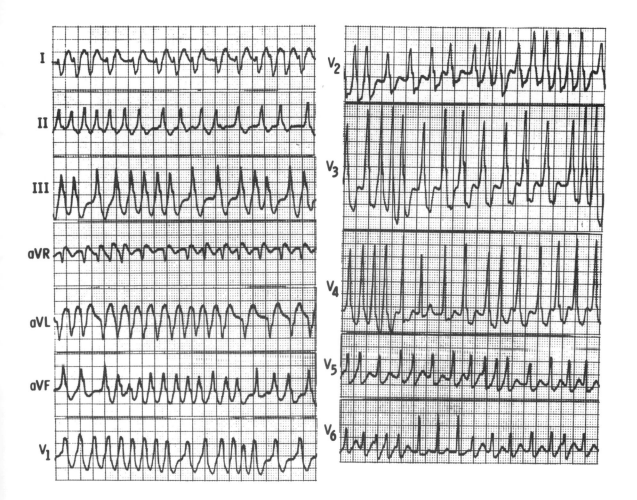

CASE 170: Diagnosis

The cardiac rhythm is AF with very rapid ventricular response (rate: 200–300 beats/min) and anomalous AV conduction. Ventricular tachycardia and even ventricular flutter or ventricular fibrillation is closely simulated because of broad QRS complexes with very rapid ventricular rate.

When the QRS complexes are extremely bizarre and when AF has a very rapid ventricular rate (ranging from 160 to 300 beats/min), the underlying disorder is almost always WPW syndrome. When this rapid heart action was terminated in this patient, his 12-lead ECG clearly demonstrated WPW syndrome, type A (not shown here).

When the clinical situation is extremely urgent, immediate application of DC shock is the treatment of choice. Otherwise, intravenous injection of lidocaine is the treatment of choice for AF or atrial flutter with anomalous AV conduction. Even after termination of AF with anomalous AV conduction, long-term oral antiarrhythmic drug therapy is essential. Under this circumstance, quinidine or procainamide by mouth is the agent of choice for many months, years, or even indefinitely, depending upon the frequency of the tachyarrhythmia.

CASE 171

This ECG tracing was obtained from a 56-year-old woman during her annual checkup. She was asymptomatic and denied any episode of rapid heart action or palpitations.
1. What is the ECG diagnosis?

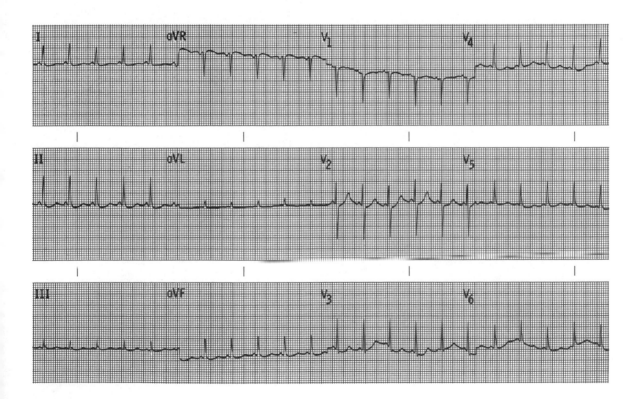

CASE 171: Diagnosis

The cardiac rhythm is sinus tachycardia with a rate of 126 beats/min. Although the P-R interval is very short, there are no other findings diagnostic of WPW syndrome. It has been shown that a short P-R interval is relatively common among healthy people (more so in young individuals), particularly during stressful situations or during physical exercise. Thus, a short P-R interval alone is insignificant clinically.

In the past, some investigators used the term "coronary nodal rhythm" to describe a short P-R interval with normal QRS complexes and normal P axis (same P axis as sinus rhythm). On the other hand, the term "LGL syndrome" has been used by others when the ECG demonstrates the short P-R interval with normal QRS complexes associated with various tachyarrhythmias.

Chapter 9
Cardiac Arrhythmias
Related to
Artificial Pacemakers

CASE 172

A demand temporary ventricular pacemaker was inserted in a 62-year-old man with recent diaphragmatic MI because of intermittent complete AV block.
1. What is the cardiac rhythm diagnosis?
2. Does the artificial pacemaker function normally?

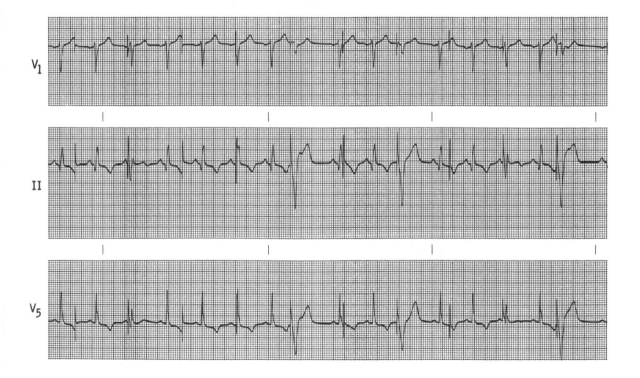

CASE 172: *Diagnosis*

The underlying cardiac rhythm is sinus with a rate of 96 beats/min. The artificial demand pacemaker functions like a fixed-rate pacemaker because of its malfunction. That is, the malfunction is a failure of sensing. Thus, the artificial pacemaker rhythm competes with the underlying sinus rhythm so that the artificial pacemaker-induced ventricular beats occur intermittently.

The diagnosis of diaphragmatic MI is obvious. In addition, posterolateral myocardial ischemia is suggested.

Manifestations of a malfunctioning artificial pacemaker include:

1. Acceleration of artificial pacing (runaway pacemaker—see Cases 182 and 183)
2. Slowing of artificial pacing
3. Irregular artificial pacing
4. Failure of cardiac capture (see Case 184)
5. Failure of sensing (see Case 172)
6. Malposition of the artificial pacemaker electrode (see Cases 177 and 180)

CASE 173

A 70-year-old woman with a permanent artificial pacemaker was seen at the pacemaker clinic at a periodic checkup.
1. What is the cardiac rhythm diagnosis?
2. What is most likely the disorder that required artificial pacing?

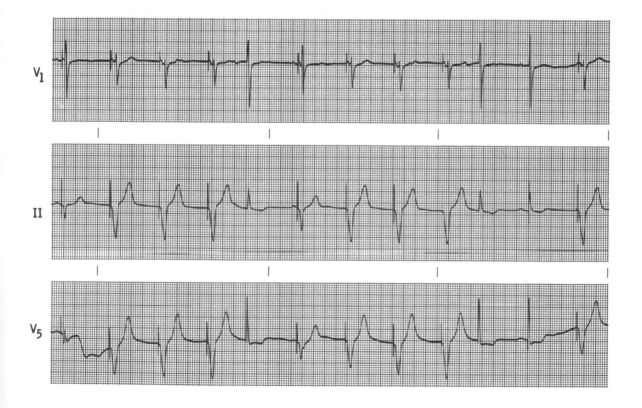

V_1

II

V_5

CASE 173: Diagnosis

The cardiac rhythm is sinus bradycardia (atrial rate: 57 beats/min) with intermittent demand pacemaker-induced ventricular rhythm (rate: 70 beats/min). Note the occasional ventricular fusion beats (the 1st and 6th beats).

The artificial pacemaker was implanted because of symptomatic SSS. Before pacing, the patient had experienced many episodes of syncope or near-syncope as a result of marked sinus bradycardia with intermittent sinus arrest and AF with advanced AV block.

The diagnosis of left ventricular hypertrophy can be made without any difficulty.

CASE 174

A temporary artificial pacemaker was inserted in a 60-year-old man with CAD because of intermittent severe sinus bradycardia.
1. What is the cardiac rhythm diagnosis?
2. What is the mode of artificial pacing?
3. What is the ECG diagnosis?

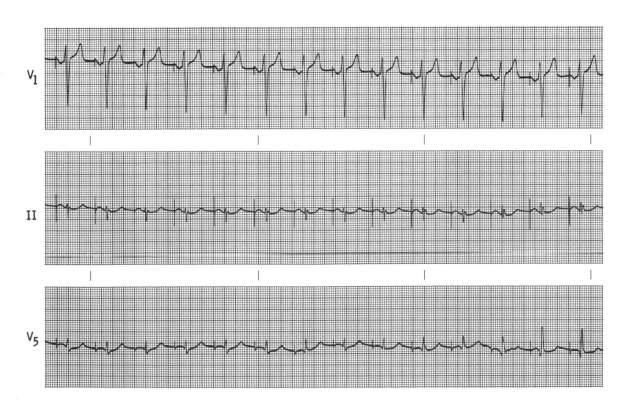

CASE 174: *Diagnosis*

The cardiac rhythm is atrial pacemaker rhythm with a rate of 85 beats/min. Note that the artificial pacemaker spikes initiate the P waves, and each P wave is followed by a normal QRS complex after a constant P-R interval.

The diagnosis of posterolateral MI can be made without much difficulty, and left anterior hemiblock is also suggested.

CASE 175

This ECG tracing was recorded on a 59-year-old man with CAD following coronary artery bypass surgery. Prophylactic artificial pacing was carried out.
1. What is the cardiac rhythm diagnosis?
2. What is the ECG diagnosis?

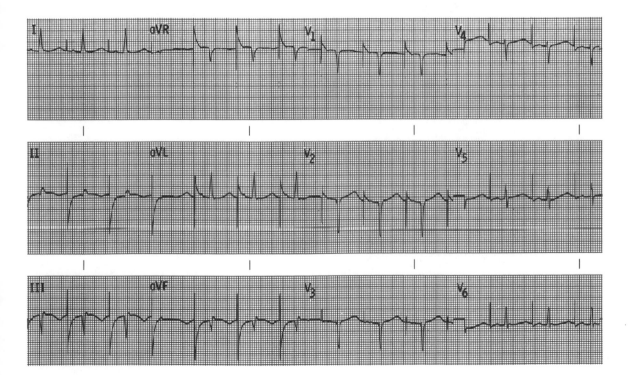

CASE 175: Diagnosis

The cardiac rhythm is coronary sinus pacemaker rhythm with first degree AV block. Note that each retrograde P wave is initiated by the artificial pacemaker spike, and a normal QRS complex follows each retrograde P wave after a constant P-R interval.

The diagnosis of diaphragmatic MI as well as anteroseptal MI can be made without much difficulty. Note the prolonged Q-T interval, which is not uncommon in patients with CAD.

CASE 176

A 61-year-old woman had received permanent pacemaker implantation about 1 year previously for the treatment of SSS. She was seen at the pacemaker clinic at a periodic medial checkup. She was not taking any medication.
1. What is the cardiac rhythm diagnosis?
2. What is the type of artificial pacemaker?

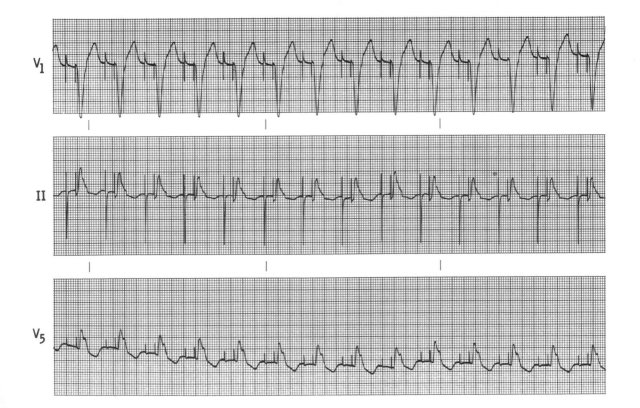

CASE 176: Diagnosis

The cardiac rhythm is AV sequential (bifocal) demand pacemaker rhythm with a rate of 90 beats/min. Note that there are 2 sets of artificial pacemaker spikes. The first spike initiates the atrial activity (P wave), whereas the second spike initiates the ventricular activity (QRS complex) with the preset P-R interval.

An AV sequential (bifocal) pacemaker consists of 2 demand units, a conventional QRS-inhibited ventricular pacemaker, and a QRS-inhibited atrial pacemaker. In this type of pacemaker, the escape interval of the atrial pacemaker is designed to be shorter than that of the ventricular pacemaker. Thus, the difference between these 2 escape intervals is a determining factor for the AV sequential delay.

The bifocal pacemaker can stimulate both atria and ventricles in sequence, or it may stimulate the atria alone or remain totally dormant. Thus, the pacemaker functions automatically according to the individual patient's needs. A bifocal pacemaker is frequently used in patients with SSS, especially when the atrial contribution is highly desired.

CASE 177

A 68-year-old man with a permanent artificial pacemaker, implanted 2 years previously, was examined at the pacemaker clinic at a routine visit. He was entirely asymptomatic.

1. What is the cardiac rhythm diagnosis?
2. Is the pacemaker working properly?

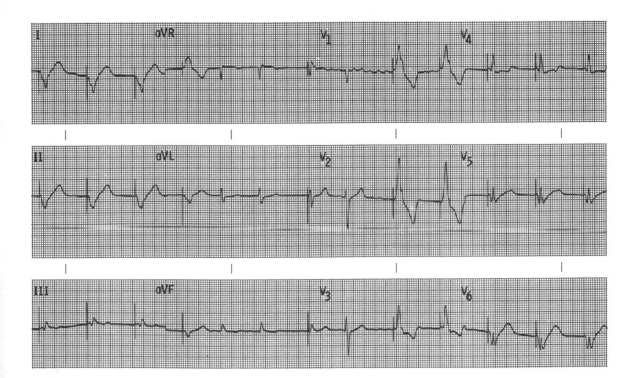

CASE 177: Diagnosis

The cardiac rhythm is atrial flutter–fibrillation with intermittent demand ventricular pacemaker rhythm (rate: 70 beats/min).

Although the artificial pacemaker functions properly as a demand ventricular pacemaker, the pacemaker electrode malposition is recognized without much difficulty. When the pacemaker electrode is situated in the expected right ventricular apex, the QRS complex of the pacemaker beat in lead V_1 should be negative (downward), whereas leads V_{4-6} (also leads I and aVL) should show upright (positive) QRS complex of the pacemaker beat. In this patient, however, the QRS configuration of the pacemaker beat is upright in lead V_1 and negative in leads I and V_6—exactly the opposite directions to those of the QRS complexes originating from the normally positioned pacemaker electrode. The above-mentioned analysis can be carried out without any difficulty using a vectorial approach.

CASE 178

This ECG tracing was obtained from an 89-year-old man with a permanent artificial pacemaker. Recently, he experienced irregular heartbeats. He was not taking any medication.
1. What is the cardiac rhythm diagnosis?
2. Does the artificial pacemaker function properly?

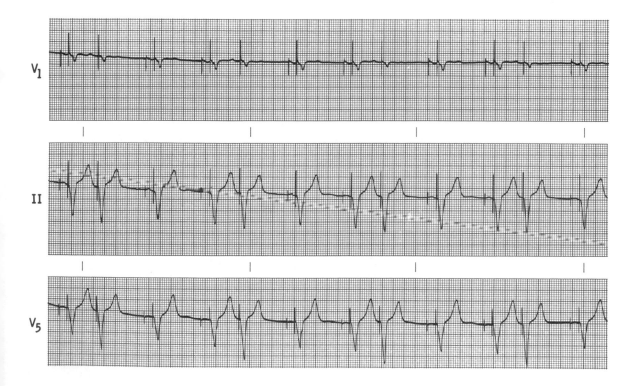

CASE 178: Diagnosis

The underlying cardiac rhythm is AV sequential (bifocal) pacemaker rhythm, but there are frequent APCs followed by the pacemaker-induced ventricular complexes. These intrinsic (natural) APCs produce atrial trigeminy, which leads to artificial pacemaker-induced ventricular trigeminy.

The above-mentioned ECG finding is suggestive of the pacemaker-sensing malfunction. Various manifestations of pacemaker malfunction are summarized in Case 172.

CASE 179

A permanent demand ventricular pacemaker was implanted 6 months ago on an 83-year-old man with complete AV block associated with several episodes of near-syncope and syncope. This is a routine ECG tracing taken during a periodic checkup. He denied any symptom.

1. What is the cardiac rhythm diagnosis?

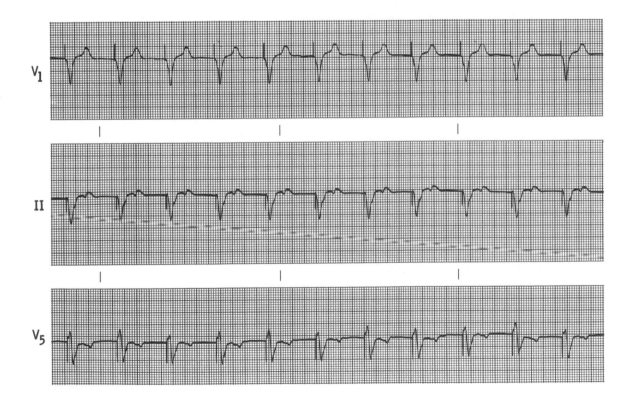

CASE 179: Diagnosis

The cardiac rhythm is artificial pacemaker-induced ventricular rhythm with a rate of 73 beats/min. It is interesting to note that each pacemaker-induced QRS complex is followed by a retrograde P wave, meaning atrial capture. The artificial pacemaker activates the ventricles and the atria sequentially throughout the tracing.

This ECG finding clearly indicates unidirectional block. In other words, this patient has complete block in forward (antegrade) AV conduction in the presence of intact retrograde ventriculoatrial conduction. It has been shown that unidirectional block is not uncommon in humans.

His permanent pacemaker functions normally.

CASE 180

Cardiac consultation was requested on a 78-year-old woman with a permanent artificial pacemaker for the evaluation of the pacemaker status. She denied any complaint.
1. What is the cardiac rhythm diagnosis?
2. What is the status of the pacemaker function?

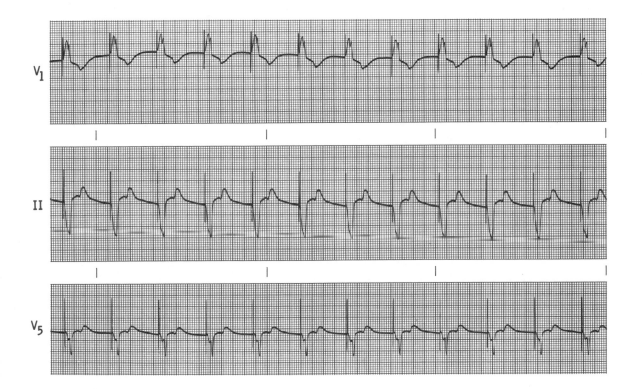

CASE 180: Diagnosis

The cardiac rhythm is artificial pacemaker-induced ventricular rhythm with a rate of 74 beats/min. Note that each pacemaker-induced QRS complex is followed by a retrograde P wave (atrial capture). This finding is a perfectly normal finding for the ventricular pacemaker.

However, the direction of the pacemaker-induced QRS complex is definitely abnormal. As described in Case 177, a normally positioned ventricular pacemaker electrode produces a negative QRS complex in lead V_1 and upright (positive) QRS complex in leads V_{5-6}. Therefore, the upright QRS complex in lead V_1 along with the negative (downward) QRS complex in lead V_5 indicates the malposition of the pacemaker electrode. In most cases, the malposition means that the pacemaker electrode is situated in the left ventricle instead of the right ventricle as a result of the penetration of the electrode through the ventricular septum. Obviously, the pacemaker electrode has to be repositioned under this circumstance.

CASE 181

This ECG tracing of a 69-year-old woman was discussed during a weekly ECG conference because of the interesting cardiac arrhythmia initiated by her artificial pacemaker.
1. What is the cardiac rhythm diagnosis?
2. What is most likely the underlying disorder that required the artificial pacemaker?

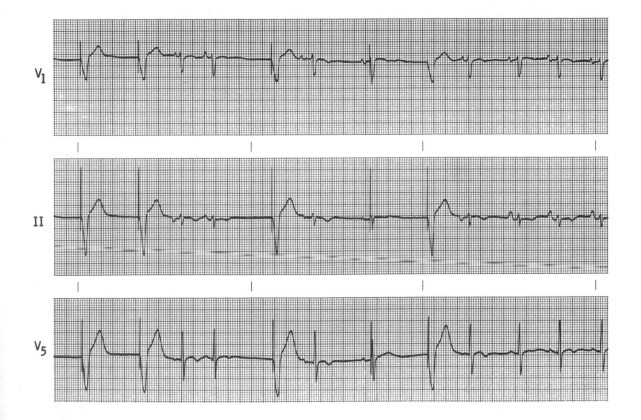

CASE 181: Diagnosis

The underlying cardiac rhythm is sinus (the last 3 beats), but a demand ventricular pacemaker takes over the ventricular activity intermittently whenever the sinus node fails to produce the cardiac impulse as a result of sinus arrest. Thus, the underlying disorder that required the artificial pacemaker is advanced SSS. Various ECG manifestations of SSS are described in Case 52.

The most interesting ECG finding in this tracing is occasional reciprocal (reentrant) beats (the 3rd and 9th beats) following the pacemaker-induced QRS complex with very long R-P interval (markedly delayed retrograde conduction). In addition, there is an atrial premature contraction (the 4th beat). Needless to say, the QRS complex of the reciprocal beat, as well as an APC, is identical to that of the sinus beat. Some P waves are deformed because they represent atrial fusion beats (the 6th and 7th beats).

Reciprocal beats occur as a result of the reentry phenomenon in the AV junction. Generally, markedly depressed conductivity in the AV junction provides the best opportunity for the production of the reciprocal beats such as are seen in this ECG tracing.

Her artificial pacemaker functions normally.

CASE 182

These cardiac rhythm strips were obtained from a 69-year-old man who had had a permanent artificial pacemaker implanted 14 months previously. He was brought to the hospital because of fast pulse rates. Leads II-a, II-b, and II-c are not continuous.
1. What is the cardiac rhythm diagnosis?
2. What is the treatment of choice?

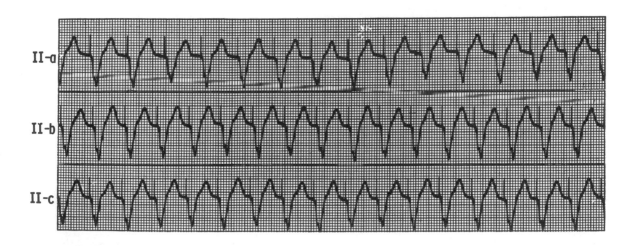

CASE 182: Diagnosis

The atrial mechanism is most likely sinus, but most P waves are not clearly evident. There is an artificial pacemaker-induced ventricular rhythm with a rate of 108–125 beats/min. It is obvious that not only is the pacing rate faster than the preset rate (60 beats/min) but also the pacing is irregular. This finding is a good example of malfunctioning artificial pacemaker. The malfunction of the pacemaker may be manifested by slowing or acceleration of the preset pacing rate. The acceleration of the pacing rate is termed "runaway pacemaker," which is almost always found in a malfunctioning fixed-rate ventricular pacemaker. Either a slowing or an acceleration of the pacing rate may be associated with irregular pacing or failure of the ventricular capture or sensing (see Case 172).

The treatment of choice is immediate discontinuation of the malfunctioning unit. This can be done by cutting the electrode wires near their attachments to the pacemaker. Connecting a temporary pacemaker to the bare electrode ends usually results in prompt recovery of most patients. A new well-functioning permanent unit should be implanted as soon as possible. The runaway pacemaker, needless to say, fails to respond to any antiarrhythmic agents.

CASE 183

A 64-year-old man was brought to the emergency room because of marked weakness associated with slow pulse rate. A permanent fixed-rate ventricular pacemaker had been implanted 19 months previously.
1. What is the cardiac rhythm diagnosis?

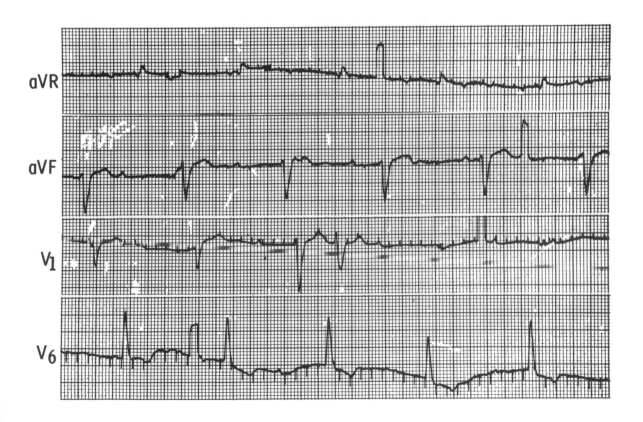

CASE 183: Diagnosis

It is obvious that there are artificial pacemaker stimuli at a rate of 490 beats/min, and all of the pacemaker stimuli fail to capture the ventricles. As a result, a preexisting complete AV block has reappeared. This ECG finding represents a far-advanced malfunctioning artificial pacemaker, termed "runaway pacemaker." Under this circumstance, immediate replacement of the unit is often a lifesaving measure.

Detailed descriptions of a malfunctioning artificial pacemaker are given in Case 172.

CASE 184

These rhythm strips were obtained from a 79-year-old man 1 day after insertion of a temporary demand artificial pacemaker for Adams-Stokes syndrome. Leads II-a and II-b are continuous.

1. What is the cardiac rhythm diagnosis?

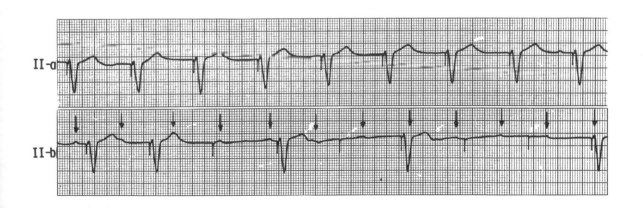

CASE 184: Diagnosis

The atrial mechanism is sinus (indicated by arrows) at a rate of 78 beats/min. Independently, there is an artificial pacemaker-induced ventricular rhythm (rate: 58 beats/min). Note the areas of ventricular standstill due to failure of ventricular capture by artificial pacemaker stimuli. This is a form of exit block. Thus, 2:1 and 3:1 exit block occurs intermittently in lead II-b.

It is very common to observe a failure of ventricular capture within 24–72 hours after insertion of an artificial pacemaker electrode, even when the electrode is correctly positioned. This form of exit block is usually transient. Otherwise, the pacemaker electrode has to be repositioned. Remember that quinidine toxicity or hyperkalemia may cause a failure of cardiac capture. Of course, far-advanced underlying heart disease may be associated with a failure of cardiac capture by the artificial pacemaker.

CASE 185

A 63-year-old woman was presented to the weekly cardiology grand rounds in view of various interesting findings, including an unusual ECG manifestation.

1. What is the ECG diagnosis?

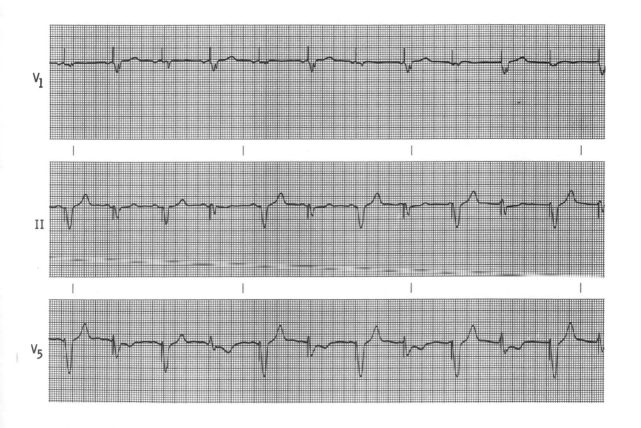

CASE 185: Diagnosis

The underlying cardiac rhythm is sinus (atrial rate: 70 beats/min), with an artificial pacemaker-induced ventricular rhythm (rate: 71 beats/min). Note that the sinus P waves and the pacemaker-induced QRS complexes are independent throughout with similar rates.

An extremely interesting ECG finding in this tracing is a variation of the QRS configuration on every other beat. The diagnosis of 2:1 ventricular electrical alternans is established. At first glance, every other beat closely simulates ventricular fusion beats.

Electrical alternans is diagnosed when the ECG complex changes its configuration at every other beat, every 3rd beat, every 4th beat, and so on. When electrical alternans involves only QRS complexes, the term "ventricular electrical alternans" is used. Electrical alternans involving only P waves (called "atrial electrical alternans"), S-T segment, or T wave is extremely rare. The term "total electrical alternans" is used when electrical alternans involves the P waves as well as QRS complexes. Again, total electrical alternans is very rare indeed. Two to one (2:1) electrical alternans (the ECG complex changes on every other beat) is the most common alternating ratio. Three to one (3:1) or 4:1 electrical alternans is rather unusual. I have observed only 1 case of electrical alternans involving only U waves. Electrical alternans associated with an artificial pacemaker-induced ventricular rhythm is also extremely rare.

In general, electrical alternans nearly always occurs in patients with advanced ventricular dysfunction or massive pericardial effusion. Ventricular electrical alternans is the most common form of electrical alternans.

Chapter 10
Miscellaneous ECG Findings

CASE 186

Cardiac consultation was requested on a 48-year-old man for the evaluation of his cardiac arrhythmia. He denied any symptoms and was not taking any medication.
1. What is the cardiac rhythm diagnosis?
2. What is the proper therapeutic approach?

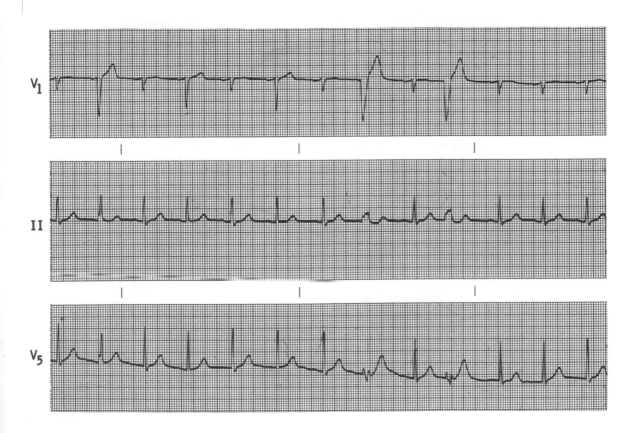

CASE 186: Diagnosis

The underlying cardiac rhythm is sinus with a rate of 82 beats/min. There are frequent ventricular ectopic beats that appear to be frequent VPCs. By close observation, however, the diagnosis of ventricular parasystole (rate: 42 beats/min) can be entertained by recognizing varying coupling intervals with constant shortest interectopic intervals and frequent ventricular fusion beats (the 2nd, 4th, and 6th QRS complexes).

It has been shown that ventricular parasystole is much more common than atrial or AV junctional parasystole (see Cases 187, 188, and 197). Parasystole is considered to be a benign arrhythmia, and no treatment is necessary.

Parasystole consists of the simultaneous activity of 2 (rarely more) independent impulse-forming centers, 1 of which is protected from the other, each competing to activate the atria or ventricles or both.

The diagnosis of parasystole is made based on these criteria:

1. Varying coupling intervals
2. Constant shortest interectopic intervals
3. Long interectopic interval showing multiples of the shortest interectopic intervals
4. Frequent appearance of fusion beats (not always present)

The usual rates in parasystole range from 40 to 60 beats/min, but parasystolic tachycardia may be observed on rare occasions.

CASE 187

This ECG tracing was obtained as part of an annual medical checkup on a 77-year-old man. He was asymptomatic and was not taking any drugs.

1. What is the cardiac rhythm diagnosis?

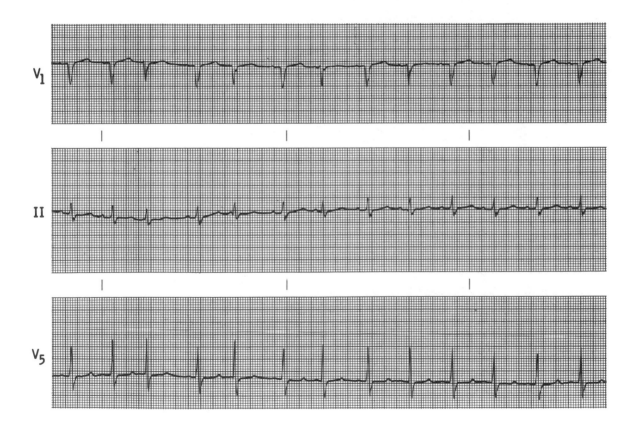

CASE 187: Diagnosis

The underlying cardiac rhythm is sinus (rate: 86 beats/min), but there are frequent AV junctional ectopic beats. The ectopic beats have the same configuration as the sinus beats, indicating that they are supraventricular in origin.

AV junctional parasystole (rate: 43 beats/min) can be diagnosed using the diagnostic criteria described in Case 186. Note that the coupling intervals vary and the shortest interectopic intervals are constant.

CASE 188

This ECG tracing of a 76-year-old man was discussed during a weekly ECG conference because his arrhythmia was thought to be somewhat unusual. He was asymptomatic.

1. What is the cardiac rhythm diagnosis?

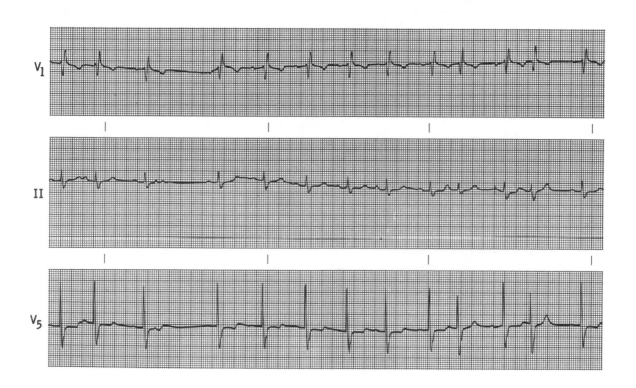

CASE 188: *Diagnosis*

The underlying cardiac rhythm is sinus (rate: 76 beats/min), but there are frequent atrial ectopic beats that superficially resemble frequent APCs. However, many experienced readers should be able to recognize that the coupling intervals vary. In addition, the shortest interectopic intervals remain constant. Thus, the diagnosis of atrial parasystole can be established without much difficulty (see Case 186). It is interesting to note that 1 atrial parasystolic P wave is not followed by QRS complex (blocked atrial parasystolic beat) because of a very short coupling interval. Of course, no treatment is necessary for atrial parasystole.

Incomplete RBBB and nonspecific S-T segment and T wave abnormality are also present in this tracing.

CASE 189

This is a routine ECG tracing of an 80-year-old woman. She complained of no symptoms.
1. What is the cardiac rhythm diagnosis?

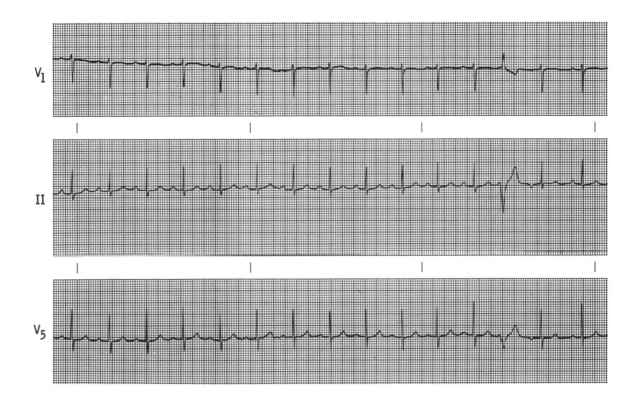

CASE 189: Diagnosis

The underlying cardiac rhythm is sinus (rate: 93 beats/min) with first degree AV block (P-R interval: 0.22 second).

There is an obvious VPC, which is followed by a retrograde P wave. The retrograde P wave occurs earlier than the basic sinus P-P cycle and represents a reciprocal beat that follows a long R-P interval after a VPC.

It has been shown that a reciprocal beat tends to occur when there is a significant conduction delay in the AV junction (either antegrade or retrograde direction) because the depressed conductivity provides the best background for the production of a reentry phenomenon in the AV junction.

CASE 190

A regular irregularity of the cardiac cycle was observed in an 86-year-old woman with mild systolic hypertension. She was not taking any medication.
1. What is the cardiac rhythm diagnosis?
2. What is the proper therapeutic approach?

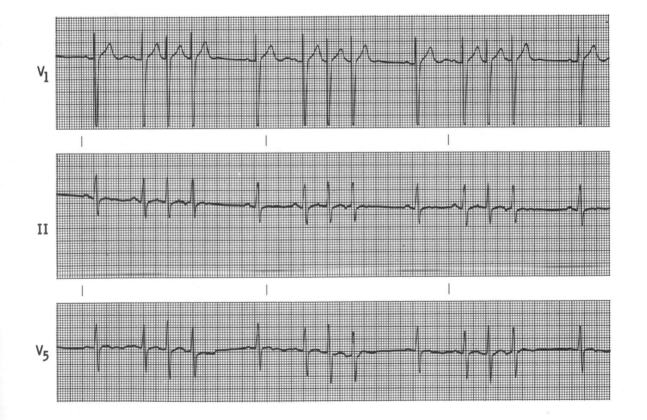

CASE 190: Diagnosis

The underlying cardiac rhythm is sinus (rate: 75 beats/min), but there are frequent APCs followed by retrograde P waves. These retrograde P waves most likely represent reciprocal beats due to a reentry phenomenon. Reciprocal beats following APCs are somewhat unusual electrophysiologic phenomena, but this ECG finding may be recognized from time to time when any physician interprets many ECG tracings on a daily basis.

A regular irregularity of the cardiac cycle is observed in this patient because APCs occur with a regular rhythmicity (atrial trigeminy), and all APCs are followed by the reciprocal beats.

No treatment is necessary under this circumstance as long as the arrhythmia causes no symptom.

CASE 191

This ECG tracing of a 66-year-old man with hypertension and COPD was presented to the weekly advanced arrhythmia conference because his cardiac rhythm was considered to be very interesting. He was not taking any medication other than hydrochlorothiazide 50 mg daily by mouth.

1. What is the cardiac rhythm diagnosis?

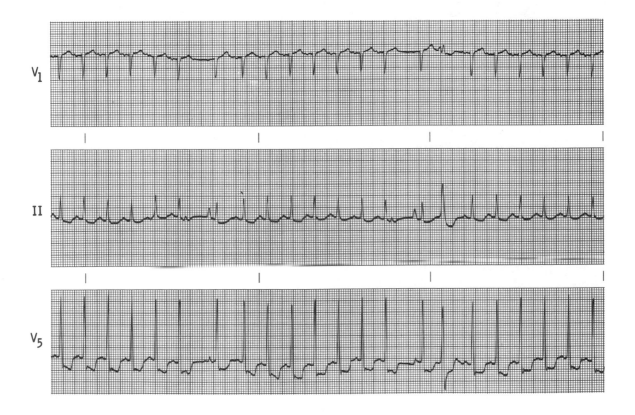

CASE 191: Diagnosis

The underlying cardiac rhythm is marked sinus tachycardia with a rate of 145 beats/min. Note 2 blocked APCs (the 7th and 16th P waves), which are followed by very tall P waves. The markedly deformed P wave most likely represents aberrant atrial conduction (Chung's phenomenon) of the sinus P wave.

Aberrant atrial conduction may be observed following a variety of ectopic beats, but this finding seems to occur most commonly following a blocked APC.

It has been shown that aberrant atrial conduction is nearly always found in elderly individuals or patients with various heart diseases. The exact mechanism for the production of aberrant atrial conduction (Chung's phenomenon) is not clearly understood, but alteration of the refractory period of the atria following a variety of ectopic beats seems to play a role. Note also a VPC.

No treatment is necessary for APCs or aberrant atrial conduction.

The diagnosis of left ventricular hypertrophy can be established in this patient without much difficulty. Marked sinus tachycardia in this patient was considered to be due to significant congestive heart failure, which was the primary reason for his admission.

CASE 192

This is a routine ECG tracing of an 81-year-old woman. She denied any symptoms and was not taking any drugs.
1. What is the cardiac rhythm diagnosis?

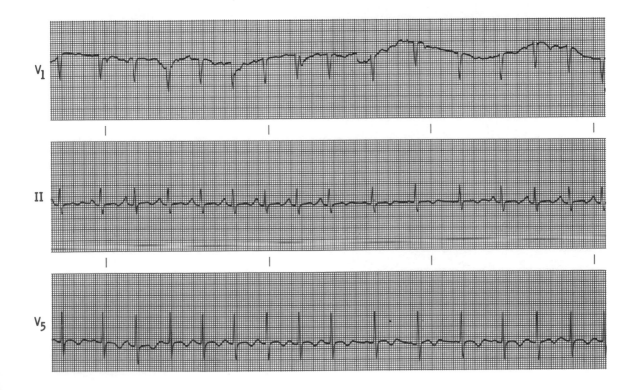

CASE 192: Diagnosis

The underlying rhythm is sinus, but the P wave configuration changes with an irregular P-P cycle. Thus, the cardiac rhythm diagnosis is sinus arrhythmia with wandering atrial pacemaker.

It has been shown that wandering atrial pacemaker is relatively common in elderly individuals, and this finding often indicates unstable sinus activity, which may be an early sign of SSS. On the other hand, wandering atrial pacemaker in children and young adults is considered to be an exaggerated form of marked sinus arrhythmia. This finding is a benign arrhythmia in this circumstance.

CASE 193

This ECG tracing was taken on a 77-year-old man with known CAD. He was not taking any medication.
1. What is the cardiac rhythm diagnosis?
2. What is the proper therapeutic approach?

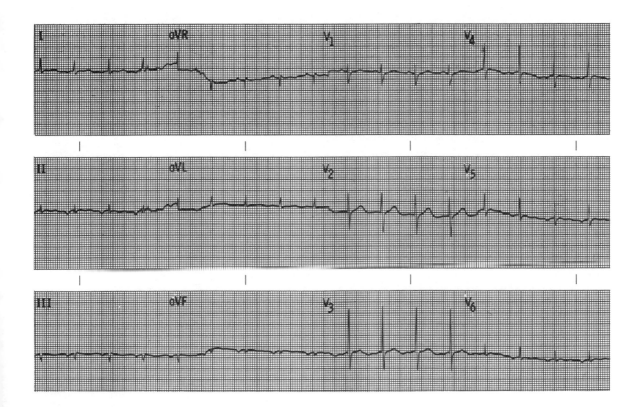

CASE 193: *Diagnosis*

Experienced readers may be able to diagnose left atrial rhythm by recognizing retrograde P waves in leads I, II, III, aVF, and V_{4-6} and upright P waves in leads aVR and V_1. Left atrial rhythm superficially resembles AV junctional rhythm or tachycardia, but an upright P wave (without any negative component) in lead V_1 and inverted P waves in leads I and V_{4-6} exclude a possibility of AV junctional rhythm or tachycardia.

The clinical significance of left atrial rhythm is uncertain, but this arrhythmia seems to be a nonspecific and benign finding. Thus, no treatment is necessary.

Old diaphragmatic posterolateral MI is strongly considered. In addition, there is a low QRS voltage in the limb leads.

CASE 194

This ECG tracing was taken on a 31-year-old man who visited the employee health center because of atypical chest discomfort. He was found to be apparently healthy and was not taking any drug.

1. What is the ECG diagnosis?

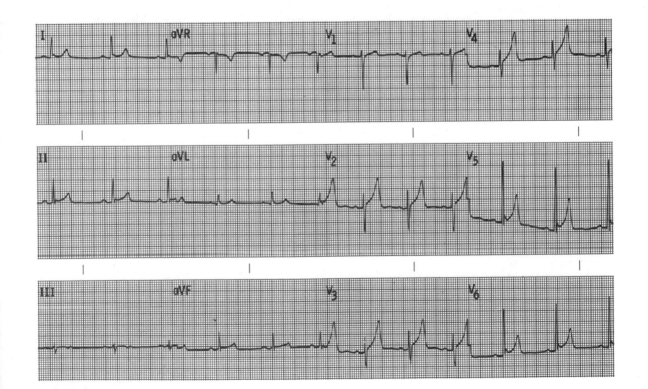

CASE 194: Diagnosis

The cardiac rhythm is sinus arrhythmia with rates ranging from 60 to 75 beats/min. In many leads (especially in leads V_{4-6}), the S-T segment is elevated, primarily as a result of J-point elevation. This ECG finding is termed "early repolarization pattern" and is a normal variant in young individuals.

The early repolarization pattern is most commonly observed among healthy black males. It superficially mimics pericarditis and at times an early phase of acute MI.

High left ventricular voltage, as shown in this tracing, is also a common normal variant in healthy young adults.

CASE 195

This ECG tracing was obtained from a 56-year-old woman with no demonstrable heart disease. She was not taking any drugs.

1. What is the cardiac rhythm diagnosis?

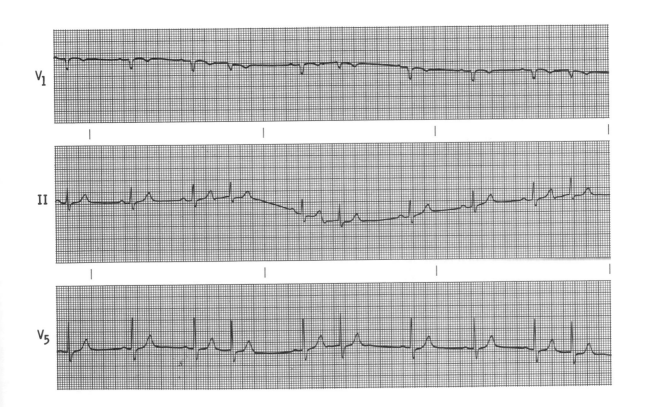

V₁

II

V₅

CASE 195: Diagnosis

The underlying cardiac rhythm is sinus bradycardia with a rate of 57 beats/min. There are 3 supraventricular premature beats, which are manifested by retrograde P waves with long P-R intervals. These ectopic beats represent either AV junctional premature contractions or reciprocal beats, although coronary sinus premature beats are also considered.

The coupling intervals vary slightly, but the diagnosis of AV junctional parasystole cannot be established (see Case 186).

CASE 196

A 65-year-old woman with CAD was evaluated at the cardiac clinic because of her arrhythmia. She was taking propranolol (Inderal) 20 mg 4 times daily by mouth.
1. What is the cardiac rhythm diagnosis?
2. What is the ECG diagnosis?

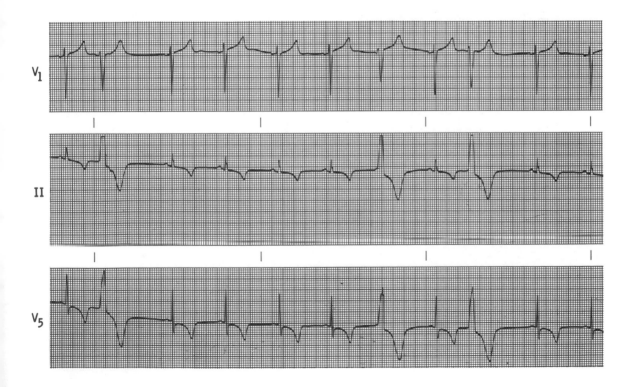

V₁

II

V₅

CASE 196: Diagnosis

The underlying cardiac rhythm is sinus with a rate of 63 beats/min. Note that there are 3 ventricular ectopic beats that appear to be frequent VPCs. However, most readers should be able to diagnose ventricular parasystole (rate: 37 beats/min) using the diagnostic criteria described previously (see Case 186), namely, the coupling intervals vary and the shortest interectopic intervals are constant.

Although ventricular parasystole is commonly found in elderly people and patients with various cardiac diseases, the arrhythmia per se is considered to be benign and self-limited. Thus, no treatment is indicated for ventricular parasystole.

Diffuse myocardial ischemia is diagnosed, and left ventricular hypertrophy is strongly considered.

CASE 197

These ECG rhythm strips of a 70-year-old man were presented to a weekly advanced arrhythmia conference because his arrhythmia was considered to be somewhat unusual. He was not taking any medication and denied any cardiac symptoms.
1. What is the cardiac rhythm diagnosis?
2. What is the proper therapeutic approach?

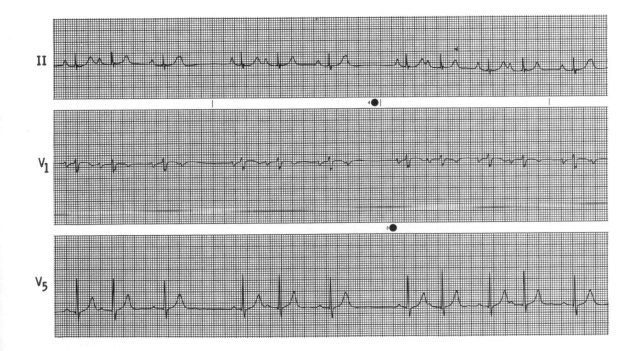

CASE 197: Diagnosis

The underlying cardiac rhythm is sinus (rate: 80 beats/min) with Wenckebach (Mobitz type I) AV block. The characteristic features of Wenckebach AV block (see Case 2) are interrupted by frequent atrial ectopic beats. The frequent atrial ectopic beats closely simulate APCs, producing atrial bigeminy. However, experienced readers may be able to diagnose atrial parasystole (rate: 42 beats/min) using the criteria described in Case 186. It should be noted that the coupling intervals vary and the shortest interectopic intervals are constant. An interesting ECG finding in this tracing is that many atrial parasystolic P waves are not conducted to the ventricles (blocked atrial parasystolic beats).

No treatment is necessary for atrial parasystole or Wenckebach AV block.

CASE 198

A 37-year-old woman with known kidney diseases was admitted to the renal service because of advanced renal failure. She was not taking any cardiac drug and was free of any primary cardiac disorder.
1. What is the ECG diagnosis?

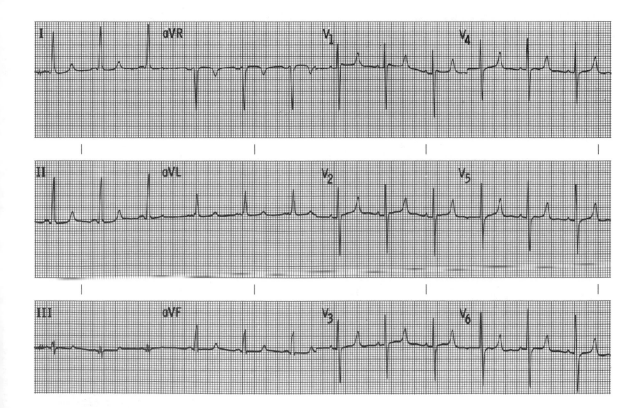

CASE 198: Diagnosis

The cardiac rhythm is sinus with a rate of 72 beats/min. There are 2 ECG abnormalities. The first diagnosis is hyperkalemia, which is manifested by tent-shaped and tall T waves with a narrow base. The second ECG abnormality is the prolonged Q-T interval as a result of the lengthening of the S-T segment due to hypocalcemia.

It has been shown that advanced renal failure is frequently associated with hyperkalemia and hypocalcemia.

CASE 199

A cardiac consultation was requested on a 57-year-old woman with breast cancer with diffuse metastases for the evaluation of her cardiac rhythm.

1. What is the cardiac rhythm diagnosis?

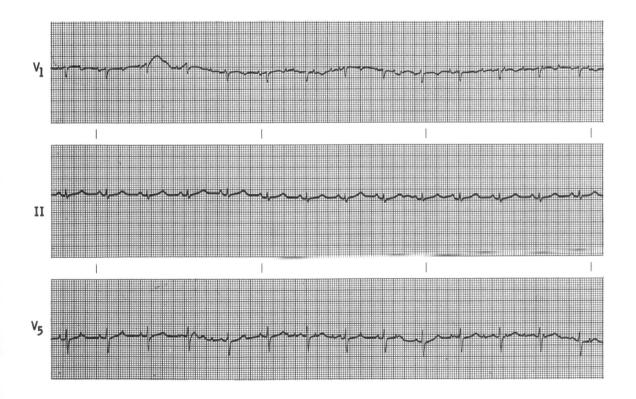

CASE 199: Diagnosis

There appear to be many ectopic P waves or atrial flutter waves, especially in leads V_1 and V_5. By close observation, however, the underlying cardiac rhythm (sinus mechanism) is not disturbed by these waves. Therefore, it becomes apparent that these waves are not true atrial activities, and they are simply artifacts.

It should be noted that various artifacts closely simulate true cardiac arrhythmias.

CASE 200

Tracings A and B were obtained from a 49-year-old woman with known congenital heart disease. Tracing A was a conventional 12-lead ECG, whereas tracing B was recorded using the right precordial leads (leads V_{1R-6R}).

1. What is the ECG diagnosis?

A

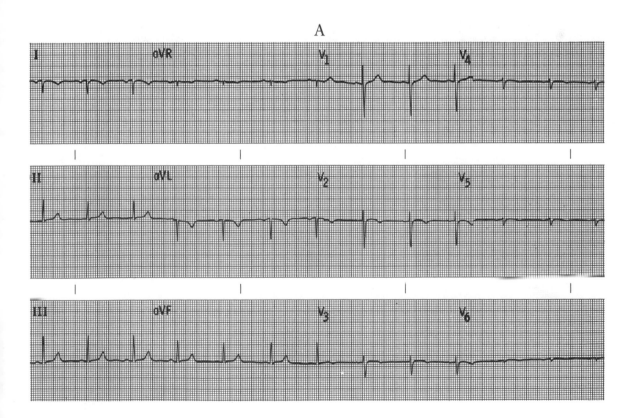

CASE 200: *Diagnosis*

Tracing A

At first glance, the electrode placement (e.g., reversed left and right arm electrodes) seems to be erroneous. However, since the precordial leads also show grossly unusual finding, it is concluded that this woman has dextrocardia.

Tracing B

When the right precordial leads (leads V_{1R-6R}) are recorded, the ECG finding is entirely normal in the chest leads.

It has been well documented that dextrocardia may be present without any other coexisting congenital cardiac defect in up to 50% of cases. Otherwise, various congenital cardiac anomalies may coexist with dextrocardia.

B

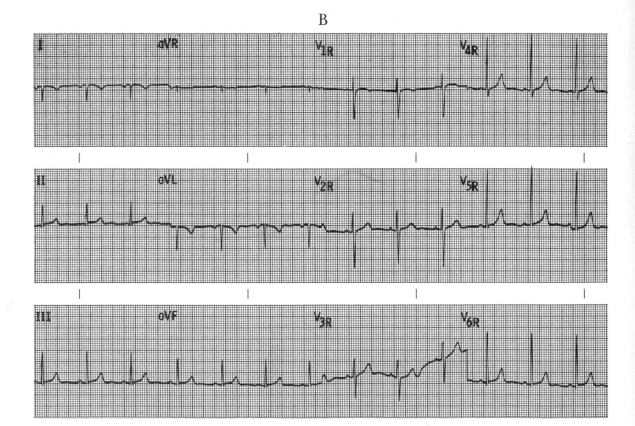